Fast Facts for the STUDENT NURSE: *Nursing Student Success in a Nutshell,* Stabler-Haas

Fast Facts for CAREER SUCCESS IN NURSING: *Making the Most of Mentoring in a Nutshell,* Vance

Fast Facts for DEVELOPING A NURSING ACADEMIC PORTFOLIO: *What You Really Need to Know in a Nutshell,* Wittmann-Price

Fast Facts for the CLASSROOM NURSING INSTRUCTOR: *Classroom Teaching in a Nutshell,* Yoder-Wise, Kowalski

Forthcoming FAST FACTS Books

Fast Facts for the OPERATING ROOM NURSE: *An Orientation and Care Guide in a Nutshell,* Criscitelli

Fast Facts for the LONG-TERM CARE NURSE: *A Guide for Nurses in Nursing Homes and Assisted Living Settings,* Eliopoulos

Fast Facts for the ONCOLOGY NURSE: *Oncology Nursing Orientation in a Nutshell,* Lucas

Fast Facts for the TRIAGE NURSE: *An Orientation and Care Guide in a Nutshell,* Montejano, Grossman

Fast Facts for the PEDIATRIC NURSE: *An Orientation Guide in a Nutshell,* Rupert, Young

Visit www.springerpub.com to order.

FAST FACTS FOR THE
MEDICAL–SURGICAL NURSE

Maggie Ciocco, MS, RN, BC, is currently a nursing program advisor for Thomas Edison State College in Trenton, New Jersey. She has over 25 years' experience in nursing education, including preceptor, mentor, staff development instructor, orientation coordinator, nursing lab instructor, and clinical instructor. Maggie received her master of science from Syracuse University, her bachelor of science in nursing from Seton Hall University, and her associate degree from Ocean County College in New Jersey. She has been an American Nurses Credentialing Center board-certified medical–surgical nurse for over 20 years. She is a member of Sigma Theta Tau and the National League for Nursing. Maggie was awarded the Sigma Theta Tau–Lambda Delta chapter Hannelore Sweetwood Mentor of the Year award in 2012.

FAST FACTS FOR THE MEDICAL–SURGICAL NURSE

Clinical Orientation in a Nutshell

Maggie Ciocco, MS, RN, BC

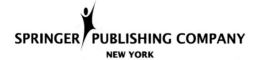

SPRINGER PUBLISHING COMPANY

NEW YORK

Springer Publishing Company, LLC
11 West 42nd Street
New York, NY 10036
www.springerpub.com

Acquisitions Editor: Elizabeth Nieginski
Composition: S4Carlisle Publishing Services

ISBN: 978-0-8261-1989-6
E-book ISBN: 978-0-8261-1988-9

14 15 16 17/ 5 4 3 2 1

The author and the publisher of this Work have made every effort to use sources believed to be reliable to provide information that is accurate and compatible with the standards generally accepted at the time of publication. Because medical science is continually advancing, our knowledge base continues to expand. Therefore, as new information becomes available, changes in procedures become necessary. We recommend that the reader always consult current research and specific institutional policies before performing any clinical procedure. The author and publisher shall not be liable for any special, consequential, or exemplary damages resulting, in whole or in part, from the readers' use of, or reliance on, the information contained in this book. The publisher has no responsibility for the persistence or accuracy of URLs for external or third-party Internet Web sites referred to in this publication and does not guarantee that any content on such Web sites is, or will remain, accurate or appropriate.

Library of Congress Cataloging-in-Publication Data

Ciocco, Margaret Curry, author.
  Fast facts for the medical–surgical nurse : clinical orientation in a nutshell / Maggie Ciocco.
    p. ; cm.—(Fast facts)
  Includes bibliographical references and index.
  ISBN 978-0-8261-1989-6—ISBN 0-8261-1989-1—ISBN 978-0-8261-1988-9 (e-book)
  I. Title. II. Series: Fast facts (Springer Publishing Company)
  [DNLM: 1. Perioperative Nursing. 2. Nurse's Role. 3. Nursing Assessment. 4. Patient Safety.
  WY 161]
  RD99.24
  617'.0231—dc23
                                                                                    2014014479

Special discounts on bulk quantities of our books are available to corporations, professional associations, pharmaceutical companies, health care organizations, and other qualifying groups. If you are interested in a custom book, including chapters from more than one of our titles, we can provide that service as well.

For details, please contact:
Special Sales Department, Springer Publishing Company, LLC
11 West 42nd Street, 15th Floor, New York, NY 10036-8002
Phone: 877-687-7476 or 212-431-4370; Fax: 212-941-7842
E-mail: sales@springerpub.com

Printed in the United States of America by Gasch Printing.

Few people in this world can truly say that they have had a lifelong dream come true—to think about it, work toward it, give it up, drop it, pick it up, examine it, and try again until finally reaching the pinnacle of success! I've been lucky enough to have that happen twice. The first time was standing on the stage at my nursing school and accepting my pin from a beloved professor. I had finally made it! The second time was publishing this book—another dream come true. The adventure will now be to realize another dream . . . what will it be?

To my husband, John, my birthday wish came true with you. Thank you for all that you do and for being there for me. You thought you would only contribute a few sentences, but this entire book would not have been written without your love, help, and support. You are my world.

To my sons, Michael and Christopher, the best gifts that I have received and truly the greatest accomplishment I've ever achieved. I love you both to the stars and back.

To P. Nicholas Ciocco—thank you for always being there, I'm so glad you chose us!

To G, J, M, and my guys . . . . thank you for loving me and giving me the strength to keep going.

Finally, to my editor and friend Elizabeth, thank you for helping make this dream come true!

"You never know what's around the corner. It could be everything, or it could be nothing. You keep putting one foot in front of the other, and then one day you look back and you've climbed a mountain."—Tom Hiddleston

I did it, Mom!!!

Contents

Part III: Must-Have Resources for the Medical–Surgical Nurse

Preface

Welcome to your new job! Whether this is your first job as a nursing professional or you are returning to the profession after an absence, please know that you are a welcome and needed resource. Behind this welcome stand those who have come before you from all over the world and from every specialty of nursing. We are all united by what made us nurses. Many of us hoped to someday model the professional behavior, skills, passion, and calm confidence of an admired professional we met during a health care encounter or in the footsteps of a loved one. No matter what brought us to the profession, we are all united in the belief that we want to help others. As nurses, no matter what area of nursing we choose, our basic goals will always be to help our patients become well, alleviate their pain and suffering, prevent disease, educate, dispel loneliness, ease birth, and comfort the dying.

While you are excited to start your first job as a nurse, you are probably nervous as well—nervous in your first care of a patient "on your own," or trying to remember the "right way" of being taught, excited for your career to start, worried you'll forget *everything,* and thrilled finally to be what you have always wanted to be! Many new nurses ask, "How long will it take for me to *feel* like a nurse?" Whether this will provide you reassurance or not, know that it will take at least a year from the start of your full-time practice for you to *finally* feel like a nurse. There will be times, more intense in the first year but continuing throughout your career, that you will feel overwhelmed, stressed out, disappointed, disillusioned, inadequate, and unintelligent—sometimes all of the above at the same time. This book has been written to not only be a practice resource but to be a comforting friend you can turn to for help and reassurance.

This text is intended to aid you in your orientation to the medical–surgical unit. It will guide you through the most common conditions seen on the unit. It does not cover or review basic anatomy and physiology or the nursing process; rather, this book is compiled from basic, time-tested, medical–surgical and subacute knowledge and best practices. In any situation, always follow the medical–surgical scope of nursing practice. It is always your responsibility to provide care within your scope and to follow your facility policies and procedures.

Chapters include a brief introduction; a focused assessment review; signs and symptoms and nursing interventions; care tips; and a feature titled "Fast Facts in a Nutshell," which provides quick summaries of important points, or those "long lost" nuggets of knowledge from nursing school or learned through hard lessons from more seasoned nurses. The final chapter is a must-have resource guide, including common pain scales; calculation guides; documentation scales for blood pressure, edema, and pulse; intramuscular technique hints; fall and restraint reduction guides; prevention of central line infection; syringe-size guides; intravenous solution review; intake and output guide; and much more.

I encourage you to see this book as an orientation review prior to your arrival on the unit and keep it handy with you as a quick, go-to resource throughout your career.

Maggie Ciocco

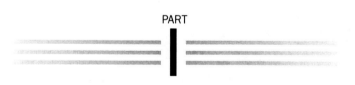

Overview of the Medical–Surgical Nursing Orientation

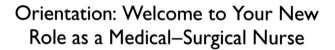

Orientation: Welcome to Your New Role as a Medical–Surgical Nurse

Orientation and preceptorship to a new unit or specialty can be a scary event to any nurse, seasoned or new. This chapter is intended to be a welcome to the profession as well as to provide basic tips for orientation. This includes understanding when you have a great (or not-so-great) preceptor, how to find a mentor, and how to take responsibility for a successful orientation.

After reading this chapter, the reader will be able to:

1. Define medical–surgical nursing
2. List five orientation tips
3. Use a preceptor checklist
4. Verbalize the difference between a preceptor and a mentor
5. List the key aspects of a mentor and list 10 key responsibilities of a mentor
6. Verbalize how to take responsibility for one's orientation and recognize when orientation is not progressing correctly

"A GOOD NURSE KNOWS WHAT SHE DOES NOT KNOW"

Pearls of wisdom can be found in many places and can inspire your nursing practice. For example, a quote from Edgar Watson Howe, an American novelist, states "a good scare is worth more to a man than good advice." For example, a medication error will cause you to remember the lesson more than any advice or instruction from your clinical instructors, professors, preceptors, or mentors.

Another pearl of wisdom referred to through years of clinical instruction is "a good nurse knows what she does not know" (Hammerschmidt & Meador, 1993). In other words, a nurse should never stop asking "why?"

- Never stop educating yourself, not only for your sake, but for the sake of your patients.
- Make sure you stay up to date in your skills and nursing knowledge.
- Ask for help when you need it, whether it is a skill you are unsure of, a patient assessment that you find troubling, or just a unit process you don't know. Your fellow professionals should not think less of you for asking questions; however, your professional integrity will come into doubt if you don't question, explore, or follow up on abnormal findings or stay abreast of current knowledge.

MEDICAL-SURGICAL NURSING

All specialty areas of nursing have their roots in medical-surgical nursing.

- Medical-surgical nursing is a specialty area of practice.
- Goals of medical-surgical nursing include assisting the patient, resident, or group in regaining or maintaining optimal health.
- Medical-surgical nurses are educators who help to prevent disease through patient education.

- The medical–surgical nurse has many skills, including assessing, diagnosing, and treating actual or potential medical conditions.
- Nursing services are provided to clients throughout the life span.
- Care is delivered in a variety of settings, including (but not limited to) acute and subacute care facilities, long-term care centers, assisted-living facilities, home care, outpatient clinics, and primary care offices.

ORIENTATION TIPS

Orientation or preceptorship is the introduction to your new career and job and may be long or short in duration. Depending on the area in which you are working, it may encompass several days of classroom learning followed by unit orientation. If you are expected to float, you may also be expected to orient on several different units. No matter the length of orientation, there are several things you can do to make your orientation as smooth an experience as possible:

Get Organized

- Know prior to your first day what type of uniform to wear or the organization's dress code, what time to show up, where to show up, and what supplies to bring.
- Many areas of nursing, particularly subacute and rehabilitation, may expect you to bring your own thermometers, blood pressure cuffs, and pulse oximeters. Question whether this is the case in your work area.
- Bring your medical–surgical text, skills book, and nursing drug book to work with you in case your facility does not have skills, policies, procedures, and other resources online.
- Complete all necessary paperwork and/or online educational offerings as required.

Review

- Review a medical–surgical text. This will help to refresh your memory on basic concepts.
- Review your nursing skills book.
- If your facility uses electronic medical records, you must still be aware of how to properly author a narrative note and what information is important to include in your documentation. Review documentation guidelines.
- Consider adding an application to your cell phone to access key references. Be aware, however, that some institutions will not allow you to access your phone during work time.

Meet and Greet

- Arrange to meet your preceptor (and some of your fellow staff) prior to the start of your orientation or work experience. When you return for your first day of work, seeing a familiar face will help to reduce your stress level.
- Take the time prior to your first day to meet with the staffing coordinator. Obtain a copy of your schedule. Negotiate for any days off you are aware of needing for preplanned vacations, school, or other circumstances.
- Seek out new learning opportunities. It can be a way to introduce yourself to other members of the team.
- Practice good communication. Be an active listener.

Take Precautions

- Inquire whether you will be orienting on the same unit and on the same shift. New nurses are often moved from unit to unit during orientation to learn in multiple areas and from multiple nurses.
- If you are moving throughout the facility during orientation, be sure that you will be with one nurse during that time on a specific unit. If you are inconsistently supervised

by your preceptor, the documented or actual outcome may not be ideal or fair.

- If your preceptor takes time off during the preceptorship, your orientation may not go smoothly. If his or her time off is excessive (say a week or more), inquire whether you may be assigned another preceptor.
- If you are off an excessive number of days, you will not have a complete orientation and may be ill prepared to work. Plan your vacation accordingly and give yourself plenty of time and opportunity to complete orientation.
- Be honest about your limitations, your skills ability, and your knowledge base. Think about enrolling in an RN refresher course prior to your job search. Make your preceptor aware of any limitations in skill level so that they can be addressed during orientation.
- Don't perform nursing care outside your scope of practice. Know your limitations with regard to what you have been taught and basic nursing practice.

A PRECEPTOR CHECKLIST

You will undoubtedly be given a checklist to have marked off by your preceptor noting the skills completed and actions taken throughout your orientation. How will you know whether your preceptor is the best one for you? It is often advisable for you to keep a checklist as well to ensure that your preceptor is ideal in her practice. Keep in mind that this is *your* orientation, perhaps your first introduction to the profession.

FAST FACTS in a NUTSHELL

A nurse's first job will be remembered long after she or he has left the position and it can affect how she or he feels about the profession of nursing. It can literally make or break him or her as a nurse.

A preceptor is ideal if she or he:

- Never leaves you alone in a new situation
- Accompanies you in all new tasks, skills, assessments, and experiences
- Completes all necessary paperwork and documentation regarding your successful (or unsuccessful) completion of the steps of preceptorship
- Provides constructive, not belittling, argumentative, or nonsupportive feedback
- Provides learning and practice objectives and experiences that are concrete and measurable
- Objectively assesses your skills
- Consistently seeks out new learning opportunities for you, introducing you to new skills and opportunities
- Introduces you to the members of the health care team and shares with you their role in the care of the patient and how they can be contacted
- Identifies areas of concern in your learning and provides additional help and teaching either herself or himself or refers you to others more qualified
- Provides you with or shows you the location of key unit policies
- Never allows you to work above your scope of practice and never allows others to ask it of you

FINDING A MENTOR

The *Oxford English Dictionary* defines a mentor as an experienced and trusted advisor. We realize that to mentor another person is a form of human development. One person is investing time, energy, and passion into assisting another person in becoming what he or she feels that person was truly meant to be.

The lucky nursing student had a professor who treated him or her as a professional long before graduation. These professors often become mentors to those new nurses. Finding a mentor may be difficult, however. What should a mentor be?

What are the key aspects of a mentor? How will you know one when you've met him or her? A mentor is above all a role model not only to you but to others in the profession. In your time with him or her, you will notice his or her interactions with others. He or she is a respected and valuable resource to not only fellow nurses but also to many members of the health care team, but what else?

- Mentors are usually the most enthusiastic and "gung ho" member of the team.
- They are the ones who think outside the box and will seek out situations to teach fellow team members.
- They actually embrace change rather than shying away from it, and see change as a way to improve patient care rather than impede it.
- They don't just punch a clock or are limited by their time at work. They work until they have completed a task or project.
- They don't horde their knowledge, but are willing to share it with their students and others.
- The mentor is also fully aware that she or he doesn't have all the answers and is continually learning. He or she continually seeks out situations in which you, as the student, can grow both in skills and in experience.
- Mentors don't shield you from situations in which you may surpass them in experience and knowledge, and aren't jealous but actually cheer you on to surpass them.

The respect you feel for your prospective mentor only grows when you see him or her in patient care situations. The mentor exudes empathy, knowledge, and patience.

The key responsibilities of a mentor are many; however, they involve many key factors. These include:

- Creating a welcoming environment for you and working to develop a rapport with you.
- Organizing and coordinating your learning activities and ensuring that learned skills take place in practice.
- Supervising you in new learning situations.
- Always acting in a professional and appropriate manner in any given situation.

- Being proud of the fact that he or she is a nurse, no matter the degree earned or specialty area worked.
- The mentor wants to share stories of success and offers helpful tips on how you can be successful as well.
- You feel comfortable asking questions, no matter whether you think they are "silly" or not. You are not belittled when you ask a question. Realize too that there are no "silly" or "stupid" questions and you should never be made to feel that you have asked one.
- You feel respected for what you can bring to a patient care situation, to your fellow staff, and to the learning environment as a whole.
- You are never made to feel uncomfortable or incompetent.
- The mentor is able to empathize with you. She or he is able to recall what it was like to be a new nurse or new employee. She or he introduces you to a new or stressful situation by letting you know that she or he was once in the same situation and understands how you feel.
- The mentor is an active listener. She or he does not assume to know your thoughts or feelings in any given situation and allows you time to express yourself.
- The mentor will be consistent and you will always know what is expected of your practice. Your goals are mutually agreed on and they remain constant.
- The mentor has shown a true desire to not only learn continually all that she or he can, but to pass that love of learning on to others.
- The mentor continually challenges you to go beyond the expected; to continually question the norm and go further than current limits, to envision the future of the profession.
- The mentor must also know that not all students and new nurses were meant to be nurses. They are not judgmental, or critical, but understand that your skills, talents, and abilities may be suited to either another specialty of nursing or to another profession altogether and will point this out to the student with care and understanding. The mentor will also guide the student to that specialty or profession in which the student may be better suited.

The list of responsibilities and characteristics of a mentor is endless because a mentor means different things to different people. It is clear, however, that a mentor is a committed professional with a passion for nursing and a true interest in furthering the profession by giving of himself or herself, his or her time, talent, and treasure.

TAKING RESPONSIBILITY FOR YOUR ORIENTATION

FAST FACTS in a NUTSHELL

When you begin your new position, take every opportunity to ensure a successful outcome.

From making sure that you will be at work on time and on all the days scheduled, to securing child care and family situations so that your mind is on orientation and not at home, *only you* can take responsibility for a quality orientation. It may happen that orientation does not go completely as you planned. You may be that new nurse who has the poor preceptor and you feel that you are not getting out of the situation all that you could. You may be part of a group of new nurses comparing notes on the progress of orientation and find that you are behind or not being exposed to as many new learning situations. You may feel uncomfortable confronting the situation, but you must take responsibility for the quality of your orientation. Document your findings using the checklist below.

- The preceptor is inconsistent in her communication with you.
- Expectations and goals are unclear, are not in writing, are not measurable, and are not achievable. Nor are they reviewed daily with you.
- You are not introduced to the team or made to feel part of the team.

- You are left alone in patient care situations, endangering both you and your patient.
- You are used as staff prior to ending your orientation.
- You are not oriented to the unit so you are therefore unclear as to where items are located and the procedures to follow.
- Your current skill and knowledge level are not ascertained prior to the beginning of orientation. Your orientation should be built on your current level of competence so that delegation is accurate.
- The preceptor does not seek out new learning experiences for you.
- The preceptor does not question you if there are areas that you feel are a weakness (i.e., a skill not experienced during clinical hours in school) and then allow you time to practice.
- He or she allows you to do the work that other staff members do not want to do.
- The preceptor is continually rude to you, fellow staff, and patients.
- He or she allows you to have a lot of down time, "hanging out" on the unit. You are not asked to partake in any care situation and made to feel like a third wheel and in the way of others.
- The preceptor frequently cancels scheduled meeting times with you and the unit educator or unit manager. This does not allow you a chance to communicate any issues.
- The preceptor allows you to find learning situations on your own; however, he or she provides guidance in the completion of a skill, assessment, or other nursing function if necessary.
- His or her clinical skills and technique are not evidence based or correct. The preceptor pressures you to perform skills as he or she does, when you are aware that to do so may bring harm to the patient.

What do you do if you are the victim of a "bad orientation"? Many new nurses are either scared to speak up because they feel it will go against them either now or later in their career in the facility, or they feel they will be fired outright. It takes courage for a new nurse (or even not so new) to be assertive in a new job situation, but it is essential. Using the aforementioned checklist as a guide, document what has occurred during your orientation/preceptorship experience.

- Ask to speak to the nurse educator of your unit or whoever is in charge of orientation. Bring your documented concerns with you.
- Avoid creating and running your own orientation in the hopes that you can salvage your experience. Your assigned preceptor must still complete documentation on your experiences and skills and this may further lead to disruption and bad feelings.
- Be professional but be assertive and state what you need in order to have a complete and thorough orientation. State what has been happening and how you feel it can be rectified. This may mean requesting a new preceptor.

If you are not satisfied after this initial encounter voicing your concerns, then you must have the courage to submit a formal complaint or grievance to your nurse educator or staff development office. Please know that formal orientation programs should provide you the opportunity to complete evaluations of not only the orientation process but of the preceptor as well, but this does not occur until the end of your preceptorship. The facility nursing department takes these evaluations seriously and will use the evaluation to adjust future orientations, perhaps to the point of not using a weak preceptor.

A poor orientation will affect your attitude toward nursing education, your fellow staff, and your career as a whole. But don't only think of how a poor orientation affects you; it also affects the patients you care for. If your orientation is poor, your care will be poor as well because you were not correctly prepared.

2

Patient Safety: From Preventing Adverse Drug Events to Infection Control

Patient safety is a key responsibility of the nurse. Patients are exposed to a variety of dangers throughout the hospital admission and the nurse is the last line of defense in preventing harm. This chapter will review the Partnership for Patients initiative that will assist you in preventing injury, prolonged hospital stay, and death caused by medication errors, infection, falls, and preventable wounds.

After reading this chapter, the reader will be able to:

1. Discuss why the Partnership for Patients was developed
2. Discuss how adverse drug events (ADEs) occur
3. Discuss six ways to prevent an ADE
4. Explain the Rights of Medication Administration
5. List the "high-alert" classifications of medications
6. Discuss how "high-alert" medications can cause harm
7. Discuss how to prevent harm when administering "high-alert" medications
8. Discuss how to prevent transmission of infection

One of the goals of orientation is to give you the skills to function safely on the unit to which you have been hired or assigned. These further sections will give you insight as to how this can be accomplished.

THE PARTNERSHIP FOR PATIENTS

In 2006 the Tax Relief and Health Care Act mandated that the Office of the Inspector General report to Congress the incidents of "never events," or those adverse patient (Medicare beneficiaries) care incidences that should *never* occur. These include:

- Medication errors
- Unmonitored side effects
- Health care–associated infections
- Surgical complications due to lack of monitoring or error
- Pressure ulcers
- Fall with injury
- Fluid volume overload
- Fluid volume deficit
- Pulmonary embolism

Medicare and Medicaid pay for the care that these patients receive due to injury and prolonged hospital stays.

The Department of Health and Human Services (DHHS) leads the effort in developing systems to improve the quality

FAST FACTS in a NUTSHELL

In 2009, $4.4 billion was spent to care for patients harmed by an adverse event. A recent study found that 13% of hospitalized Medicare patients experienced an adverse event that resulted in injury, permanent harm, or death. Half of these were considered preventable.

of health care that Americans receive. The Centers for Medicare and Medicaid Services (CMS) works under the auspices of the DHHS. The CMS developed the Partnership for Patients initiative in 2011.

════════════════════════════════════*FAST FACTS in a NUTSHELL*

The goals of the partnership are to make hospital care safer, more reliable, and less costly by helping to achieve approximately 1.8 million fewer injuries to patients and saving over 60,000 lives over 3 years.

The Partnership has identified 10 core patient safety areas of focus, many of which will be discussed in this text. These include:

- ADEs
- Catheter-associated urinary tract infection
- Central line–associated bloodstream infection
- Injuries from falls and immobility
- Obstetrical adverse events
- Pressure ulcers; surgical site infection
- Venous thromboembolism
- Ventilator-associated pneumonia
- Preventable readmissions

ADEs AND HOW TO PREVENT THEM

Consider the following statistics:

- A 2013 article in *Scientific American* noted that medication errors are considered the third leading cause of death behind heart disease and cancer.

- According to the Institute of Medicine (IOM) there are 400,000 *preventable* drug-related injuries per year (an average of one error per day) in hospitals.
- 1.5 million people are harmed by medication errors every year (IOM).
- The average annual cost in the United States of medication-related injuries is $3.5 *billion*.
- These statistics do not include the number of medication errors that are *not* reported.

FAST FACTS in a NUTSHELL

> ADEs can not only cause permanent disability and death, but they also erode the trust that our patients place in us.

Medication errors occur for a variety of reasons, from lack of knowledge regarding the medication, to being interrupted during med-pass, to failures of a drug-dispensing system as a whole. The most common causes of medication errors, according to the American Society of Health–System Pharmacists, include the following:

- Confusing strength designation on medication labels
- SALADs, or "sound alike, look alike drugs"
- Equipment failure or malfunction (i.e., intravenous [IV] pumps)
- Illegible handwriting
- Improper transcription
- Inaccurate dosage calculation
- Inadequately trained personnel
- Inappropriate abbreviations used in prescribing
- Labeling errors
- Excessive workload
- Lapses in performance (interruptions, phone calls, call lights)
- Unavailability of medication

The recommendations for physicians, pharmacists, pharmaceutical companies, and hospitals on how to prevent medication errors are extensive. Nurses, however, are the last line of defense in error prevention . . . so how can *you* prevent a medication error?

- Be familiar with all policies and procedures regarding medication administration in your facility. This includes medication order processing and administration times.
- All medication orders should be verified before a medication is administered.
- ALWAYS check the original order prior to administering the first dose of a medication.
- DO NOT administer the medication unless you understand *why* you are giving the medication and that the order is correct.
- DO NOT borrow medications from another patient or other patient care unit. If an ordered medication was not sent, do not circumvent the pharmacy and administer by borrowing. There may be a reason the medication was not sent (i.e., drug allergy or other contraindication). Call the pharmacy to investigate.
- Always question when large volumes (more than two of a tablet, capsule, vial, or amp) are to be administered.
- Always understand how to use medication administration devices (i.e., IV pumps) prior to using them. Never use them without understanding how they work.
- Always, always, always STOP administering a medication when a patient questions what you are giving them. Ninety-nine times out of 100 he or she is correct that a medication is unfamiliar. Always check the original order.

FAST FACTS in a NUTSHELL

At the beside, the tried-and-true method of preventing a medication error is to follow the Rights of Medication Administration and to never deviate from them, no matter how stressed or short of time you may be.

THE RIGHTS OF MEDICATION ADMINISTRATION

The original five rights have increased over the years. The rights include:

- **The right patient**
  - Identify the patient using the facility-approved method. This can include a combination of two identifiers, such as full name and birth date, picture, or bar code system. Check the patient's FULL name against the med sheet/medication administration record (MAR) and original order.
- **The right medication**
  - Check the medication label against the original order.
  - Check the medication against the order at least three times: When removing the medication from the dispensing system, when pouring the medication, and prior to administering the medication.
- **The right dose**
  - Check the order and confirm that the dose is correct (use a drug reference manual or computer application if necessary).
  - If you must calculate a dosage, have another nurse also calculate the dose to be sure it is correct. In many facilities this is policy; if not so in yours, do it anyway.
- **The right route or the right form**
  - Check the order against the med sheet/MAR and confirm that the route is correct.
  - If the patient is unable to take the medication via the ordered route, see whether the route or type of medication can be changed.
  - NEVER crush a medication that should not be crushed.
  - NEVER mix medications together to expedite the administration process in a patient with a G-tube.
- **The right time**
  - Make sure the ordered times correspond with facility policy. Giving a medication too late or too early is a medication error.

- If giving a PRN (*pro re nata*, or as needed) medication, confirm when the last dose was given and that you are giving the dose within the appropriate time.
- Ensure that you are administering the medication on the correct date.
- **The right documentation**
  - Do not presign for medication. Sign for a medication only *after* it is given.
  - Do not wait, however, until the end of the shift to sign for medications given or to enter this information in the electronic medical record. This will prevent inadvertent double dosing of the patient by either yourself or another nurse.
  - If necessary, make sure to also include any other vital information having to do with the administration. For example, site given, laboratory value (i.e., international normalized ratio [INR]), or vital signs (i.e., heart rate or blood pressure).
- **The right reason**
  - Know the rationale for the medication you are giving. Familiarize yourself with the patient's history and why the medication is ordered.
  - If the patient's current condition or history is not compatible with the ordered medication, question the order.
  - Know *why* you are giving the medication and its desired (and adverse) effects. If you are not knowledgeable, seek answers through drug literature or the pharmacist on staff.
- **The right response**
  - After giving the medication, determine whether the desired response was achieved. For example, after giving acetaminophen for a fever, did the patient's temperature decline?
  - After giving pain medication, was there a relief or reduction in pain?

Document the response of the patient to the medication and other nursing interventions. If the response is not appropriate or not reached, report it.

MEDICATION RECONCILIATION

Effective communication among the patient and family, physician, nurse, and facility is also important in preventing ADEs. Many facilities have implemented various methods of reconciliation, including collecting a list of patient medications on admission. This list should be compared to the physician-ordered medications. When transferring the patient to either units within the facility or another health care facility, compare the list of home medications, current medications, and medications to be taken on facility discharge (i.e., to long-term care [LTC] or subacute). Clarify all orders with the physician.

HIGH-ALERT MEDICATIONS

High-alert (or high-hazard) medications are those medications that, even when used correctly and no error in administration has occurred, still have the potential to cause significant harm to the patient. When an error does occur with the medication, the impact on the patient has the potential to be major. The Institute for Healthcare Improvement (IHI) recognizes four groups of high-alert medications because they "represent the areas of greatest harm and greatest opportunity for improvement." The types of harm that can occur with these medications include hypotension, bleeding, hypoglycemia, delirium, lethargy, and oversedation. The high-alert medications include:

- Anticoagulants
- Narcotics and opiates
- Insulins
- Sedatives

Anticoagulants can cause harm because, although they are widely used, their management is not consistent. The effects of warfarin (Coumadin) can be altered by interaction with food and medications both prescribed and over the counter. Lab results of INR may not be reliable. Correct anticoagulant management of patients before and after surgery is also difficult to achieve. Patients may be at risk of either bleeding or blood clots, both due to ineffective monitoring.

Narcotics and opiates: Effective pain control is an essential part of patient care because patients need to have their pain controlled in order to recover from injury, surgery, and illness. Those patients with chronic pain require effective pain control in order to fully function for as long as possible. Patients may be at risk of harm from narcotics even when they are ordered and dispensed correctly. Harm can include:

- Oversedation
- Respiratory depression
- Confusion
- Lethargy
- Nausea
- Vomiting
- Constipation

Much of the prevention of harm with narcotics lies with appropriate drug ordering by the physician or health care provider. Inappropriate monitoring of the patient and lack of communication by the nurse can lead to overdose, underdose, respiratory depression, and poor pain control. Even when a patient receives patient-controlled anesthesia (PCA), thought to lead to decreased narcotic issues, harm can still occur due to drug interactions, inappropriate use of the PCA by the patient, and PCA malfunction.

Insulins are difficult to regulate in those patients who are stressed from illness and surgery, who are undergoing procedures, or those who have not had adequate food/caloric intake. Even when closely monitored in the before-mentioned circumstances, the patient can suffer from hypoglycemia/hyperglycemia.

Sedatives are a necessary part of procedures that patients undergo. When used inappropriately, sedatives can lead to oversedation, hypotension, delirium, and lethargy (contributing to fall). Nurses and physicians can both contribute to the harm of the patient if they are not aware of the onset of action of sedatives. Many physicians do not follow the adage to "start low and go slow" when ordering original and increasing doses. Facilities may have inadequate processes to address emergency situations caused by sedatives, such as respiratory depression and arrest.

Many facilities have protocols and systems in place to eliminate the effects of high-alert medications. You, as the nurse, can prevent harm from high-alert medications by adhering to the following guidelines:

- Adhere closely to the rights of drug administration previously mentioned.
- Closely follow and adhere to order sets, preprinted order forms, clinical pathways, protocols, and policies.
- Read and adhere to all warnings regarding medications.
- Include parameters for the medications that require them. Examples include blood pressure for hypertensive medications or INR levels for warfarin. Know the expected parameters of the medications you are administering. If parameters are not given by the MD, request them.
- Follow drug precautions posted by the pharmacy either directly on the medication or by some other means of communication.
- Check lab work *prior* to administering medications that require lab monitoring.
- Educate the patient regarding the action of the medication and its side effects and when to contact you or the MD should there be an issue.
- Know the protocols for "rescue" of the patient. Examples include those patients suffering from hypoglycemic reactions and oversedation.
- Attend all education having to do with medications. Contact staff education if you feel you need additional instruction.
- Read labels carefully.
- Make sure IV pumps are working correctly. Manually check infusion settings with your calculations. Have another nurse perform the calculations as well.
- Be familiar with dosage levels and recommendations of medications.
- Follow guidelines for vital sign monitoring while the patient is on the medication.

UNIT SAFETY

When you begin to work on your new unit, you need to familiarize yourself with the various locations of patient safety equipment. This includes the following:

- The automated external defibrillator and crash cart
- Know the location of emergency preparedness and disaster manuals.
- Fire exits and fire extinguishers; know your role in the event of a fire on your unit
- Know all the emergency codes (fire, disaster, elopement, cardiac arrest, medical emergency, rapid response, in-house security issue, bomb threat, and so on). Know your role in each of these events.
- Know the location of Material Safety Data Sheets manuals and follow guidelines for using any chemicals in your work area.
- Know how to properly report an incident. Many facilities allow all personnel to complete online reporting that is sent directly to facility risk management.

INFECTION CONTROL

Nearly 1 in every 20 patients acquires an infection during his or her hospital stay. The IHI has addressed four major infections, including catheter-associated urinary tract infections, central line–acquired bloodstream infections, postoperative infections, and ventilator-associated pneumonias. These will be addressed in later chapters.

In 2007 the Healthcare Infection Control Practices Advisory Committee published recommendations for health care facilities and guidelines as to when their employees should apply isolation precautions. These measures protect patients, staff, and visitors from being exposed to infectious agents. There are two types of isolation precautions—standard and transmission based. Standard precautions advise that you should assume that every patient you come into contact with has an infectious disease that can be passed on to you or other patients. Because it is not always known who has an infectious disease, you have to take precautions every time, with every patient. Standard precautions include:

- **Hand hygiene.** Wash your hands following Centers for Disease Control and Prevention (CDC) guidelines. Hand washing (instead of alcohol gel) should be used when hands are visibly dirty, after you use the restroom, and before eating or preparing food. Adhere to CDC guidelines for using alcohol-based hand rubs as well. Perform hand hygiene before and after each patient contact, after touching anything in the patient environment, before and after a patient care procedure, and after removing gloves.

- **Personal protective equipment (PPE).** This is equipment or clothing that is used by staff to protect them from infection or injury. This includes face shields, masks or goggles, gloves, and gowns/aprons. PPE is proactively worn prior to performing a patient care task that may expose you to blood or body fluids. Wear the correct PPE every time you enter an isolation room and at other times when it is required.

- **Patient care equipment.** Use single-use equipment in an appropriate manner. Don't share patient equipment. Wear gloves when handling equipment that is visibly soiled and perform hand hygiene after handling. Follow facility guidelines when cleaning soiled patient care equipment. If the sterility of a package has been compromised, don't use the product.

- **Environmental cleaning/disinfection.** Follow facility guidelines for the care and cleaning/disinfection of environmental surfaces, particularly those in the patient area.

- **Patient placement.** Appropriately communicate if your patient develops an infection that can be transmitted to others due to poor hygiene, wound drainage, vomiting, or diarrhea. Be aware of when your patient is at risk for infection as well and take precautions.

- **Handling of laundry.** Don't place soiled linen on the floor in patient care areas, don't carry linen close to your body, wear gloves when handling soiled linen, and don't store clean linen in a patient room. Don't agitate or shake out linen in a patient care area (i.e., when making a bed).

- **Safe injection practices.** Follow facility policy regarding the use of its needleless system. Always be aware of and use safety features. Never recap, bend, break, or manipulate used syringes. Keep used sharps in view at all times prior to disposal. Dispose of used sharps in puncture-resistant containers and follow guidelines for when these containers should be changed.
- **Resuscitation practices.** Never perform mouth-to-mouth resuscitation during cardiopulmonary resuscitation. Use a mouthpiece or Ambu bag.
- **Respiratory hygiene/cough etiquette.** Instruct your patients and, if necessary, their visitors to cover their mouth/nose when coughing or sneezing (into their arm, not their hand). Instruct them on the proper disposal of tissues. Instruct both to perform hand hygiene after using tissues.
- **Safe lumbar procedures.** Ensure that physicians and those assisting them wear a surgical mask when inserting catheters or injections into the spinal or epidural space.
- **Additional tips.** Wear only a plain wedding band; rings with stones harbor bacteria. Maintain the closed system of urinary catheters and IV lines; follow facility guidelines when cleaning IV, peripherally inserted central catheter (PICC), and central line sites; use aseptic technique when required, such as when inserting a Foley catheter; be aware of when you break aseptic technique; police yourself as to when to stop a procedure and begin again following proper technique.

The second tier of infection control is transmission-based precautions. This goes above and beyond the standard precautions that are used for all patients. There are three types of transmission-based precautions: contact, droplet, and airborne. Follow facility guidelines for patient placement under the appropriate precautions and the PPE that should be worn in each.

FAST FACTS in a NUTSHELL

A health care–acquired infection is the most frequently reported adverse event in health care.

3

Nursing Assessment Basics: Focused Assessment and the PQRST System

In an ideal situation, a complete head-to-toe assessment would be conducted for each patient by each nurse that cares for the patient. Time constraints and patient acuity, however, often exclude this type of assessment. You will be completing shorter, more focused assessments throughout the admission of the patient based on chief complaint or current abnormality of the patient. Skills to be reviewed in the chapter also include communication between health care professionals.

After reading this chapter, the reader will be able to:

1. State when a focused assessment should be completed
2. Use the "PQRST" system
3. List 10 assessment techniques
4. Use the "SBAR" technique
5. List phone skills to use when speaking to other health care professionals

INITIAL ASSESSMENT

When you admit a patient to your facility, you will complete a thorough health history. This assessment is the beginning of your nursing process. Remember to always introduce yourself and explain your purpose before beginning to gather information.

The health history will include:

- Current and past medical history, including childhood illnesses
- Chronic illness/disease: onset, duration, signs and symptoms, and management
- Acute illness/disease: onset, duration, frequency, signs and symptoms, and management
- Family history (cause of death of immediate family members, medical condition of family members)
- Social support (psychosocial aspects of care)
- Immediate and past surgical procedures
- Previous major injuries
- Current treatments
- Immunizations and tuberculosis status
- Cognition, behavior, and mood
- Communication ability
- Hearing
- Vision
- Diet and nutrition (including presence of enteral feedings and swallowing ability)
- Oral cavity assessment
- Bowel and bladder evaluation
- Skin evaluation and pressure sore risk assessment
- Fall risk predictor assessment
- Pain evaluation
- Current medications (including over-the-counter medication and illicit drugs)
- Use of alcohol and tobacco
- Allergies, including those to drugs and food, and the reaction that occurs

Included in the health history is a general review of body systems with very general questions asked of the patient. It is the responsibility of the nurse to follow up with more focused questions if an issue or problem is noted. If the patient is unable to give a complete history, the family or significant other may be asked to help complete the history.

The second part of the health history includes a physical assessment. On transfer to either another unit (i.e., medical–surgical to the intensive care unit) or to another facility (i.e., hospital to subacute or long-term care), another physical assessment will be completed and it should be compared to the baseline obtained by the prior unit or facility.

A FOCUSED ASSESSMENT

In an ideal situation, a complete head-to-toe assessment would be completed for each patient by each nurse who cares for him. Time constraints and patient acuity, however, often exclude this type of assessment. You will be completing shorter, more focused assessments throughout the admission of the patient based on the chief complaint or current abnormality. A focused assessment collects relevant information pertaining to the current condition of the patient after a change or new symptom develops. For example, if a patient is admitted with a respiratory issue, then a focused respiratory assessment would include vital signs; oxygen saturation; skin color; mental status; lung sounds, noting any adventitious sounds; the recognition of shortness of breath and/or edema. It is obligatory that a focused assessment be completed:

- When there is a change in the condition of the patient
- When there is a deviation from baseline in any of the body systems
- After an incident (i.e., a fall)

A focused assessment:

- Allows you to identify actual or potential patient problems
- Assists you in evaluating the effectiveness of treatments, medications, and nursing or medical interventions

The initial patient assessment enables you to develop an appropriate plan of care. The results of a focused assessment can lead to refinement of the care plan and introduction or elimination of interventions. If during your complete or focused assessment you notice anything not within normal limits or a deviation from the baseline, begin to question the patient. For example, if during the respiratory-focused assessment discussed before you notice the patient has shortness of breath, ask the patient whether he has experienced this before. The focused assessment together with direct questioning helps you to concentrate on vital information that needs to be further explored and possibly reported.

FAST FACTS in a NUTSHELL

The four assessment techniques include inspection, palpation, percussion, and auscultation. They are always completed in this order except in the instance of a gastrointestinal assessment, in which case it is completed as inspection, auscultation, percussion, and palpation.

THE PQRST SYSTEM

Use the "PQRST" system to guide your data collection and to determine what questions to address to the patient. A set of vital signs, including oxygen saturation, should also be obtained concurrently. After ascertaining the patient's primary complaint, begin the "PQRST." Ask open-ended questions of the patient and your subjective documentation should be in the words of the patient. If your patient's symptoms are or become life-threatening, remember your ABCs (airway, breathing, circulation) and assess those immediately.

The "PQRST" system was originally developed as a pain assessment tool, but has been modified to address *any* patient complaint. The letters stand for lines of questioning used to investigate a patient's experience or symptoms.

- P = Provocative/Precipitating/Palliative
  - Aggravating factors
  - Associated symptoms
  - Alleviating factors—what makes the signs and symptoms worse (breathing, coughing, moving)?
  - What makes them better?
  - Does your palpation make the symptoms worse or better?
  - Do medications make it better (note the medications)?

- Q = Quality or Quantity
  - What do the signs and symptoms feel like?
  - How often has this occurred?
  - Objectively, what do the sounds and symptoms look like or sound like to you as the nurse?
  - Has this symptom ever happened before now? Is this time worse than last time?
  - How does this symptom affect the patient's normal activity, or activities of daily living (ADL)?

- R = Region, Radiation, and Related Symptoms
  - Where in the body is the symptom occurring?
  - Is the symptom moving to another part of the body?
  - Have the patient point to where the symptom is occurring.
  - Does the complaint/problem relate to another issue? For example, if the patient has pain in the lower abdomen, is it accompanied by nausea or fever?

- S = Severity
  - Is the symptom becoming worse, better, or staying the same?

- How does this symptom affect the patient's normal activity, or ADL?
- Rate the symptom on a scale of 0 to 10. (This type of scale works well in measuring symptoms of nausea, dyspnea, pain, or other subjective complaints.) However, use your discretion and critical thinking to determine whether the patient report is accurate.

- T = **Timing** (history, onset, frequency, duration)
  - When did the complaint/symptom begin?
  - Was the onset sudden or gradual?
  - How often does the symptom occur, and when it does, how long does it last?
  - Is the symptom better, worse, or different from onset?
  - How long has it been since onset?

- U = **Understanding** (added to the basic PQRST system by some health care agencies)
  - What does the patient think caused the pain?
  - Can the patient relate the pain to anything (i.e., muscle pain with lifting something heavy, or chest pain after exercise)?

ASSESSMENT TIPS FOR THE BEGINNING OF YOUR SHIFT

Organizing the beginning of your shift can take some time to perfect. This depends on your training and the areas you have previously practiced and lessons learned in the past. Each patient care situation will teach you where to focus and what should be your priority.

Before Getting Report

- Check orders written in the past 24 hours and any orders or treatments that need to be carried out on your shift.
- Check schedules for therapy and surgery. Are preop medications scheduled? Do your patients require pain medication prior to therapy? Are there treatments that must be completed prior to your patient leaving the unit?

At the Bedside

- Introduce yourself to the patient and explain what you are doing. Provide for privacy.
- Check your patient after getting report. Briefly assess the patient's orientation and general state and stability. Ensure that there are no immediate problems.
- If a problem or issue is noted, address it immediately before continuing. Small problems tend to snowball into larger ones.
- Complete either a focused or more thorough head-to-toe assessment on your patients. Begin with patients that may be leaving the unit for a test, therapy, or surgery.
- Know that when you are speaking to your patient you are also assessing mental status, skin color, breathing effort, and facial symmetry.
- Part of your assessment should include anything "attached" to the patient. This includes intravenous lines (IVs), enteral feedings, Foley catheters, chest tubes, suctions, drains, wound vacs, and so on. Make sure that all monitors, pumps, specialty beds, and other machinery are working correctly. If not, find out why and attempt to correct the situation.
- Make sure that intravenous solutions are correct and infusing at the correct rate. Ensure that enough solution remains until you are available to change the bottle. Make sure the pump is plugged in or charged. If it is your facility policy, zero out the total infused on IV and enteral feeding pumps so that it begins at "0" for your shift.
- Trace lines and tubing back to the patient and assess insertion sites, noting any signs of inflammation and infection.
- The output of your patient is also part of your assessment. Note the amounts of suction, urinary drainage, wound drainage, and so on. Note amount, consistency, odor, and color.
- Look for patterns.
- Perform a safety check. Place the call light in reach, bed in lowest position, side rails up.
- Place patient belongings in easy reach of the patient (glasses, tissues, phone, and water).

- Make sure the floor is not cluttered and any wires do not pose a tripping hazard.
- Look at the big picture. Abnormal findings need to be taken into perspective with the rest of your assessments and results.
- Compare the asymmetry/symmetry of the body (i.e., the face, or the chest while breathing).
- Compare one side of the body to the other (i.e., one leg to the other if edematous, one hand to the other if swollen, one pulse site to the other if weak or absent).

After Checking All Patients

- If patients are stable, check the medication administration record for the medication schedule for your shift.
- Document your findings.
- Communicate your findings.

FAST FACTS in a NUTSHELL

Make it a habit to follow the same system every day or you may potentially miss an important finding.

COMMUNICATION AMONG HEALTH CARE PROFESSIONALS

In 2004 a study by the Agency for Healthcare Research and Quality found that 70% to 80% of medical errors are related to communication issues. The Joint Commission on Accreditation of Healthcare Organizations (JCAHO) estimates that 63% of sentinel events occur because of poor communication. Many instances of poor communication result in patient injury and death. A 2005 study by the JCAHO found that 70% of preventable hospital mishaps occurred because of communication breakdowns. Other studies, based on this one, have shown that half of those breakdowns occur during patient "handoffs." Handoffs occur when one health care professional reports to another at either change of shift or transition of care (transfer from unit to unit or facility to facility), change of shift from nurse to nurse, or communication between physicians.

One method used to reduce the incidents of missed communication is the SBAR technique. Developed by the U.S. Navy, the SBAR method was adopted by the health care industry in the 1990s. SBAR stands for:

- S—Situation—What is happening at the present time?
  - Begin by identifying yourself and your location.
  - State the patient's name and the problem you are calling about.
  - Verbalize that you have assessed the patient and have discovered changes in the patient's status.

- B—Background—What are the circumstances leading up to this situation?
  - State a brief history and current symptoms.
  - Include neurological, cardiovascular, respiratory, gastrointestinal, genitourinary status, current lab work (compare to past lab work if relevant; i.e., current hemoglobin/hematocrit levels to previous or current drug levels to previous), current medications, and IVs if pertinent.

- A—Assessment—What is your basic assessment of the patient?
  - State what you think the problem may or may not be.
  - State whether the patient is deteriorating.
  - If the patient is unstable, state what action must be taken.

- R—Recommendation—What are your recommendations to the MD or other health care professional?
  - What should we do to correct the problem? I request that you . . . (transfer to critical care; come see the patient; order lab work, other tests, medications).
  - If the patient does not get better, when should you recontact the MD?

Remember to read back recommendations and new orders.

It is noted that new nurses consider SBAR an organizational tool. It assists them in charting and focusing on what is important in the care of the patient. It assists them in communicating patient needs to the physician.

PHONE SKILLS

After you have gathered your assessment information, and if necessity warrants, the information must be communicated to the appropriate health care provider. Never mind about a patient crashing or coding, oftentimes one of the most stressful and daunting tasks to a nurse, new or seasoned, is speaking on the phone with a physician.

Here are some tips:

- In order to build your confidence, practice what you are going to say with your preceptor prior to making a call.
    - Write down what you want to say or use a blank SBAR form.
    - Even if you are not the nurse calling, make your preceptor aware of an instance when a call to an MD should be made and practice what you would say if you were the one to make the call.
- Listen on the phone while your preceptor calls an MD. Note the information she or he provides and her or his interaction with the MD.
- While on orientation allow your preceptor to listen on the line while you are making your call. The preceptor can fill in information you miss by prompting you or speaking herself or himself, and can also critique your telephone skills.
- Always identify yourself, the patient, and your facility when making a call to any MD, health care facility, testing facility, and so on.
    - Because the individual you are speaking to may not be familiar with the patient (i.e., a covering MD), always ask "Do you know this patient?" or "Are you familiar with this patient?"
- As an RN you may be asked to call an MD for another nurse.
    - Always thoroughly investigate a situation before calling the MD.

- You may be caught off guard with questions to which you don't have the answers. Always know current medication and treatment orders, read the most recent interdisciplinary notes, and know current test results.
- It may be best to receive a mini "report" from the nurse asking you to call so that you are familiar with the case.

• Knowing when or under what circumstance to call an MD comes with experience. If you are unsure whether a call should be made, ask your preceptor, charge nurse, unit manager, or a nurse you have a relationship with on the unit first.

• Document that you made a call to an MD or other health care professional.

- Note the time and with whom you spoke and orders that were given (or if no orders were given).
- If you have had to make multiple calls and have left messages with a service or office and have not spoken to the MD, note this as well.
- Be aware of how many times you must call an MD and are not able to speak to him or her before you contact the nursing supervisor or other superior who will direct you up the chain of command.

• Have all the information you need prior to calling an MD. Try not to place an MD or any other health care professional on hold while you scramble to obtain necessary information.

• If you encounter a rude MD or other professional, don't retaliate by being rude yourself.

- Be calm and polite.
- State what you need to say in order to obtain a necessary order for your patient or to provide needed information.
- Remember, you are a patient advocate and information must be shared in order to provide quality care for the patient.
- If an MD or any other professional is rude to you, report him or her to your nurse manager or supervisor.

Common Medical–Surgical Conditions and Emergencies

4

Neurological Deficits in the Medical–Surgical Patient: Altered Mental Status Can Occur in Any Patient

The neurological assessment for the medical–surgical nurse is less in depth than that of a nurse working in critical care. However, no matter what specialty worked, a neurological assessment is an essential part of the nursing exam. Any patient, regardless of diagnosis, can experience a neurological deficit. The early recognition of a neurological event can help to impact positively the outcome for the patient. Evaluation of level of consciousness (LOC) and mentation are the most important parts of the neurological exam.

After reading this chapter, the reader will be able to:

1. Explain the care of the patient experiencing a seizure
2. Explain the care of the patient experiencing a stroke
3. List the symptoms of altered mental status (AMS)
4. List the items to be documented in a patient with seizure
5. List types of common headaches

FAST FACTS in a NUTSHELL

A change in LOC or mentation is usually the first clue to a deteriorating neurological condition.

For every patient you encounter, your neurological assessment should begin when you walk into the patient's room. When you engage your patient in conversation, you are assessing his or her orientation, speech, facial symmetry, mood, affect, and cognition.

You should perform a more focused neurological assessment if the patient experiences:

- Pain (headache, backache, extremities). Note the onset (sudden, gradual), frequency, duration, and character (throbbing, achy, dull, sharp). Note whether the pain radiates and whether it is precipitated or relieved by any factors. Be aware of any trauma in the patient's past medical history (i.e., head injury). Note any related symptoms, such as nausea or spasms.
- Dizziness or vertigo
- Lightheadedness/faintness
- Loss of consciousness
- Visual disturbances
- Motor/sensory loss or complaints

A FOCUSED NEUROLOGICAL ASSESSMENT

A focused assessment should be based on the patient's diagnosis and the presenting problem if you notice a deficit. Compare the patient's current LOC, mental status, thought process, and motor and sensory function to the baseline, and note any change from baseline. Is the symptom or finding occurring on one side of the body, that is, is it unilateral or bilateral?

- Determine the chief complaint.
- Be aware of your patient's past medical history, including seizures; head trauma; headaches; hypertension; diabetes, infections; tumors; and alterations in the cardiac, renal, and hepatic systems.
- Be aware of current medications, as neurological issues can be caused by combinations of medications or side effects of medications.
- Be aware of allergies.
- If the patient is able to speak, ask whether the onset of the complaint was gradual or sudden, or whether it was preceded by an aura (a subjective complaint of an odor, light flashes, or air movement) that can occur at the onset of a migraine or seizure.
- Inquire whether the patient was aware of what may have caused the event.
- If there is pain, describe the character. If a headache is present, have the patient rate the pain. For example, is this the worst headache the patient has ever had, or has he or she had this pain before?
- Note the time and duration of the complaint.
- Note the patient's mental and cognitive status, beginning with LOC.
- Determine the patient's affect or mood. Does the patient appear or act agitated, calm, restless, irritable, argumentative, labile, detached, sad, or indifferent? Is the mood or affect appropriate for what is happening or for the environment?
- Determine the patient's behavior. Is the patient anxious, agitated, crying, depressed, using slowed movements, or overexcited (manic)?
- Determine the patient's cognition. Note whether the patient's thought processes, content, and reasoning have changed from baseline. Is the patient having delusions or hallucinations? Is he or she acting paranoid?

- Determine whether the patient is having new difficulty with grooming or personal hygiene. This can be the result of a motor deficit or onset of brain disorder or emotional or psychiatric disorders.
- Note the patient's speech and language. If the patient had been able to speak, is speech now difficult (dysphasia) or absent (aphasia)? If the patient is unable to speak or write his or her thoughts, the patient has expressive aphasia. If the patient's speech is clear but not related to the questions asked, then this is termed *receptive aphasia*. If the patient has lost both the ability to speak and to understand, it is termed *global aphasia*.
- Determine the patient's orientation to person, place, time, and situation.

COMMON NEUROLOGICAL DISORDERS SEEN ON THE MEDICAL–SURGICAL UNIT

The most common neurological issues that develop on a medical–surgical unit include the following:

- Altered mental status
- Headaches
- Stroke
- Seizure

Altered Mental Status

AMS is the most common neurologic emergency. It can occur in hospitalized patients due to hypoxia, hypoglycemia, head injury, an infection in the brain, brain tumor, psychological condition, or a metabolic alteration or as an adverse effect of medications.

Be careful when describing a patient's AMS. Describing terms can be confusing to multiple professionals because they themselves may not be clear as to their meaning. Instead of using a specific term, describe how the patient responds to verbal and physical stimuli.

For clarification, listed below are the terms used to describe AMS:

- Full consciousness = patient is alert, attentive, and follows commands. If awakened or already awake at time of exam, the patient remains awake.
- Lethargy = patient awakens easily but not fully and remains drowsy. The patient answers questions appropriately but follows commands slowly.
- Obtunded = patient is difficult to arouse and requires constant verbal and/or physical stimulation to remain awake and follow commands. The patient may slowly respond to a simple question, but gives confused answers. The patient falls back to sleep between verbal or physical stimulation.
- Stupor = patient only arouses to some type of constant, usually painful stimuli. Painful stimuli may only elicit a moan and an attempt to withdraw from the stimuli. Commands are not followed.
- Coma = patient does not respond to any type of stimulation. There is no movement except for some reflexes. There is no verbal response.

Hypoglycemia nearly always causes an alteration in mental status and decreased LOC. Moderate hypoglycemia affects the central nervous system because it deprives the brain cells of fuel. Signs and symptoms include inability to concentrate, headache, lightheadedness, confusion, memory impairment, irritability, altered vision, combativeness, and drowsiness.

If hypoglycemia is not corrected, it can become severe and cause disorientation, seizures, and loss of consciousness. Nursing interventions for patients with AMS include:

- Obtain vital signs, including blood glucose level.
- Monitor the patient's ABCs (airway, breathing, and circulation) and ensure that your patient is breathing and has a patent airway. Patients who have AMS from a stroke can lose their airway quickly or stop breathing.
- Monitor the patient's blood pressure and heart rate, noting the strength and rhythm. If the heart rate is low and the blood pressure is high, it could indicate intracranial bleeding.
- If there is no pulse, initiate cardiopulmonary resuscitation.
- Ensure that there is a patent intravenous site in order to provide any ordered fluids or medication.
- Assess for any internal bleeding that could be causing hypovolemia, for example, if the patient is postoperative or is prescribed anticoagulants.
- Note any obvious causes for the AMS by completing a neurological assessment.
- Use a facility-approved stroke scale to determine whether the patient's AMS is being caused by a stroke. These scales usually include determining the patient's ability to smile (facial droop), move his or her arms (palms up and no drift of one or both arms or hand grip), and verbalization (clearly with no slurring, or the ability to speak at all).
- Note whether the patient suffered a seizure.
- Suction as needed.
- Provide supplemental, high-flow oxygen. Monitor the patient's oxygen saturation.

Headache

Headaches are the most common neurological complaint. They can be a symptom of a serious disease or a condition all its own. A headache that is severe and with sudden onset requires rapid assessment and intervention. This type of headache is associated with hemorrhagic stroke, brain tumor, and meningitis.

The majority of headaches, however, are not a medical emergency. These include tension, migraine, and sinus headache.

- Tension headaches are the most common and they are caused by muscle contractions in the head and neck. These are attributed to stress. The pain is described as squeezing, dull, or achy.
- Migraine headaches are believed to be caused by contraction of the blood vessels. The pain is described as pounding, throbbing, or pulsating and is often associated with visual changes.
- Sinus headaches are caused by fluid pressure inside the sinus cavities of the face and skull. They are often accompanied by nasal congestion, cough, and/or fever.

Be prepared to report the headache if it is sudden and severe and/or accompanied by fever, seizures, or AMS. Nursing interventions for headaches include:

- Rest in a quiet environment
- Consider and provide nonpharmacological measures to reduce the pain, such as cold cloths to the forehead
- Administer analgesics and monitor for effectiveness
- For migraines, consider oxygen therapy

Stroke

The third leading cause of death in the United States is stroke or cerebral vascular accident. A stroke occurs when there is a disruption of blood flow to the brain resulting in a loss of brain function. It is more common in the geriatric population. Strokes can occur in either the left or right side of the brain. The symptoms that the patient displays will indicate the side of the brain where the event has occurred. Risk factors include high blood pressure, heart disease, diabetes, cigarette smoking, and prior stroke. There are two types of stroke:

- Ischemic stroke: These are the most common, accounting for 80% of strokes. Ischemic stroke results from an embolism or thromboembolism in blood vessels leading to the brain. The usual cause is atherosclerosis.

- Hemorrhagic stroke: Accounts for 10% to 20% of strokes. It results from bleeding inside the brain and is usually fatal. Risk factors include hypertension, stress, or exertion. The most common symptom is a sudden, severe headache.

Signs and symptoms of a stroke must be reported immediately. Treatment with tissue plasminogen activator must be started within 3 hours of initial symptoms in order to prevent long-term or permanent neurological defects. Signs and symptoms may include:

- Facial drooping, tongue deviation
- Sudden numbness or weakness in the face, arms, legs, or one side of the body
- Pupils may become unequal, either becoming dilated or fixed on the affected side of the brain
- Sudden, severe headache
- Sudden loss of vision in one eye or sudden onset of blurred or double vision
- Difficulty swallowing
- Decrease in LOC
- Speech disorders, slurred speech, difficulty speaking or understanding speech
- Inability or decreased ability to move an extremity
- Sudden loss of balance or difficulty walking, dizziness, or weakness. Patient may state one side of the body feels "dead"; lack of muscle coordination
- Disturbance in taste or smell
- Altered LOC exhibited by combativeness, restlessness, lethargy, apathy, or confusion

FAST FACTS in a NUTSHELL

Patients who are experiencing a transient ischemic attack (TIA) have the same symptoms as those who are having a stroke. In a TIA the symptoms may gradually decrease within minutes; however, they still require complete medical evaluation. It is a medical emergency and may be a sign of an impending stroke.

The medical condition of the stroke victim may deteriorate quickly. The patient will require continued ongoing assessment. Nursing interventions include:

- Maintaining a patent airway; supporting the ABCs
- Applying oxygen to reduce hypoxemia and monitor the pulse oximetry
- Monitoring respiratory rate and type; alterations may be noted due to brain damage.
- Monitoring blood pressure. Fluctuations in blood pressure may indicate cerebral pressure or damage to the vasomotor area of the brain. Take blood pressure readings in both arms and compare. Artery blockage may be demonstrated by different readings.
- Noting trends in alteration in LOC; is it stable or decreasing?
- Noting and reporting signs of intracranial pressure; these include symptoms of altered LOC, including restlessness, confusion, and irritability. There may also be changes in speech, pupillary reactivity, heart rate, headache, nausea, vomiting, and alterations in vision
- Turning the patient on the *affected* side so that secretions can drain from the mouth.
- Noting pupil reactions; the pupil size, shape, equality, and light reactivity are affected by damage to the cranial nerves.
- Elevating the head, but not flexing the neck; this reduces arterial pressure and improves blood circulation to the brain.
- Protecting paralyzed extremities
- Maintaining verbal communication with the patient; the patient may retain the ability to understand even when he or she is unable to speak.
- Preparing the patient for transfer to the intensive care unit

Seizure

A seizure is a sudden, abnormal electrical discharge from the brain that results in changes in sensation, behavior, movements, perception, or consciousness. A seizure can occur due to low blood glucose, fever (usually in younger patients), poisoning, drug or alcohol withdrawal, or traumatic brain injury. It can also occur without history of disease or disorder. Seizure can occur at any time of life either with or without warning and may become chronic. Causes of seizures can be divided into six categories:

- Cerebral pathology—recent or old head injury, stroke, infections in the brain, hypoxia, brain lesions, brain tumors, delirium, Alzheimer's disease, and increased intracranial pressure
- Toxic agents—poison, alcohol, drug overdose, chronic alcoholism
- Chemical imbalance—hypoglycemia, hypokalemia, hyponatremia, hypomagnesemia, renal failure, hypoxemia, and acidosis
- Fever—heatstroke, infections
- Eclampsia
- Idiopathic—unknown origin (epilepsy)

There are two major classifications of seizures. This is based on electroencephalographic findings and seizure type.

- **Partial (focal) seizure**—occurs in a limited part of the brain
  - Most common type
  - Further classified according to whether consciousness has been impaired; partial and complex
  - *Simple* (partial motor, partial sensory). A specific part of the brain is involved, so then a specific part of the body is affected. For example, the seizure may manifest itself as a jerking of the hand or a fixed gaze. Consciousness is not impaired, but the patient cannot control what is happening.
  - *Complex*—the patient loses consciousness
- **Generalized (formally, grand mal) seizure**—involves both hemispheres of the brain
  - Comprises one third of seizures
  - Patient loses consciousness
  - May or may not convulse

- When convulsions occur they involve all body muscle groups.
- Includes absence, myoclonic, clonic, tonic, tonic–clonic, and atonic seizures

Seizures of any type that last more than 30 minutes are termed *status epilepticus,* and are a life-threatening medical emergency. The most frequent seizure seen in the hospital is the generalized tonic–clonic seizure. Seizures occur in three phases: prodromal or preseizure, in which the client may experience an aura; ictal, or the seizure; and postictal, the period following the seizure. Symptoms of a generalized seizure include:

- Loss of consciousness
- Hypertension, tachycardia, sweating, and intense salivation
- May be convulsive or nonconvulsive
- Dilated pupils
- Stridorous breathing, excessive salivation
- Incontinence
- Postictal: exhaustion, sleepiness, weakness, confusion, amnesia concerning the seizure, possible nausea, sore muscles

Symptoms of a partial complex seizure include:

- Patient remains conscious
- Possible reactions, such as like a dream state, staring, wandering, irritability, hallucinations, uncontrollable fear
- Involuntary motor symptoms, such as lip smacking
- Purposeful but inappropriate movements
- Antisocial behavior
- Postictal phase—no memory of the seizure, confusion

Symptoms of a partial simple (focal–motor/Jacksonian) seizure include:

- Preceded by an aura
- No loss of consciousness if unilateral or loss of consciousness if bilateral
- Convulsive movements and disturbance of the body part controlled by the brain involved (i.e., parietal lobe

involvement = numbness or tingling, occipital lobe involvement = bright, flashing lights)

Please note that, if observed, all preseizure signs and symptoms should be documented. These include:

- If there were stimuli to the seizure; these include visual, auditory, olfactory, and tactile stimuli. Also note whether the patient complained of psychological or sleep disturbances.
- Note whether the patient complained of an aura.
- Note where in the body the seizures or movements began, the direction of the eye gaze, and the position of the head. These all give clues to the location in the brain where the seizures occurred.
- Movements of the body parts and areas of the body involved
- Whether the patient's eyes were open and pupillary reaction
- Whether the eye and/or head was turned to one side
- The presence or absence of involuntary muscle activity, such as lip smacking and eye blinking
- Whether the patient was incontinent
- Duration of the seizure
- If the patient lost consciousness and, if so, for how long
- If the patient is able to move his or her arms and legs after the seizure
- If the patient is able to speak after the seizure
- Whether the patient was confused after the seizure
- If the patient slept after the seizure

Nursing Care of the Seizure Patient

Nursing care of a patient experiencing a seizure includes:

- Padded side rails, bed in lowest position
- Strict bed rest if patient verbalizes signs of an aura; remove dentures or any food from the mouth
- Remain with patient during and after seizure.
- Turn patient to the side on a flat surface and suction as needed to prevent aspiration.

- Loosen clothing from around neck and chest.
- Follow facility policy regarding use of bite blocks and airway insertion.
- Do not restrain the patient. If seizure occurs when the patient is out of bed, lower patient to the floor, ensuring the head is cushioned.
- Perform neurological assessment, including vital signs after the seizure.
- Reorient the patient as needed.
- Administer medications as ordered.
- Administer oxygen as needed postictally.

5

Assessment Skills to Differentiate Signs and Symptoms of a Cardiac Event From Other Possible Conditions

Patients may have a history of cardiac disease and are on your unit for treatment. Other patients may be admitted with a noncardiac-related issue and develop a cardiac emergency. In either case, your assessment findings and immediate action are necessary in order to prevent harm. You need to be able to see the "whole picture" of the patient and understand that signs and symptoms of cardiac disease may mimic other causes.

After reading this chapter, the reader will be able to:

1. List symptoms of a myocardial infarction
2. Perform a focused cardiac assessment
3. Perform a chest pain assessment
4. List interventions for venous thromboembolism
5. List interventions for chest pain

CARDIAC ASSESSMENT BACKGROUND

A cardiac assessment should be completed on a patient with a known cardiac disorder who is admitted to your unit. However, you can objectively determine when a cardiac assessment should be completed at other times based on what you encounter when you speak with your patients. Are they having difficulty breathing? Is their color pale or cyanotic? Do they seem anxious?

You should perform a more focused cardiac assessment if the patient experiences:

- Complaints of chest pain or discomfort and/or unrelieved epigastric distress
- Shortness of breath or difficulty breathing
- Sudden onset of stomach upset, nausea, or vomiting together with sweating (diaphoresis)
- Anxiety and irritability, or if he or she verbalizes a feeling of impending doom
- Increased or slowed heart rate from baseline
- A feeling of heart "skipping beats" (palpitations)

FAST FACTS in a NUTSHELL

NEVER ignore a patient (or family member) when he or she tells you "something isn't right" or "I'm going to die!" Nine times out of 10, the patient will be coding within minutes to hours of uttering that statement. ASSESS, ASSESS, ASSESS and closely monitor the patient. It is a phenomenon all seasoned nurses have seen, no matter their area of practice.

A FOCUSED CARDIAC ASSESSMENT

On encountering any patient that you suspect may be experiencing a cardiac issue, you should immediately perform a focused assessment. Compare all findings to baseline and note any change. Included in this assessment should be a set of vital signs, including blood glucose and pulse oximetry. Note the rate and character of the respirations and pulse. Include a mental status check and note the patient's skin color and other objective changes.

- Note any personal or family history of cardiac disorders, hypertension, coronary artery disease, and lung disease.
- Note any cardiac medications and their expected and adverse side effects. If the patient states that he or she has stopped the medications, inquire as to why (i.e., "makes me cough" or "gives me indigestion"). Follow up with an MD.
- Is the patient able to care for himself or herself and perform his or her normal activities?
- If the patient is complaining of chest pain, refer to the section following on chest pain.
- If the patient is having shortness of breath (dyspnea), ask if this has happened before and what brought it about. Does the shortness of breath change with position, come and go suddenly, or interfere with the patient's activities of daily living (ADL)?
- If the patient is coughing, note frequency, severity, and cause, if known or as described by the patient. If sputum is produced, describe the quantity, color, and odor. Note if it is blood-tinged.
- Note any new complaints of fatigue or whether the patient tires easily.
- Observe the body as a whole. Are there signs of edema, cyanosis, pallor, or any other skin changes? Note the location and whether it is unilateral or bilateral. What makes any of the signs better or worse (i.e., swollen feet subside after putting the legs up)?
- Does the patient have to get up at night to urinate? Is this a new occurrence?

Physical Exam

- Note whether the jugular veins are distended. This is achieved by observing the patient sitting at a 45-degree angle in the bed.
- Auscultate the carotid arteries; the presence of a bruit indicates a blockage in the artery.

> Ask the patient to hold his or her breath while you auscultate for bruit. The breath sounds can often be confused with bruit.

- Palpate the carotid arteries (never at the same time). Note the strength. The pulse should be the same bilaterally.
- Inspect the patient's skin color and note any lesions, absence of hair, sores, bruising, or rash.
- Note the warmth, color, and moisture of the skin. Color is an important indicator of blood flow:
  - Pallor seen at the fingernails, lips, and oral mucosa indicates decreased arterial blood flow or anemia.
  - Redness in the feet while dependent may mean chronic arterial insufficiency.
  - Peripheral cyanosis of the lips, ears, extremities, and nail beds may mean decreased blood flow due to constricted arteries. May be seen in heart failure.
  - Central cyanosis of the tongue and buccal mucosa is more serious and can mean pulmonary edema.
- Auscultate the blood pressure.
- Palpate the peripheral arteries. They should be equally bilateral. If a pulse is weak or absent, use a Doppler device to auscultate. Follow facility-approved protocol for marking the location of the pulse for future assessment purposes. Document and report weak or absent pulses.
- Auscultate the heart sounds, noting any adventitious ones.

FAST FACTS in a NUTSHELL

> Never auscultate a blood pressure on the arm that has an intravenous line, or on the side of a patient who has had a mastectomy, arteriovenous fistula, or shunt. Repeat with a manual cuff if abnormal. If abnormal, repeat the assessment in both arms.

COMMON CARDIOVASCULAR DISORDERS SEEN ON THE MEDICAL–SURGICAL UNIT

The most common cardiovascular disorders and emergencies seen on the medical–surgical unit include the following:

- Chest pain
- Heart failure
- Angina pectoris
- Myocardial infarction
- Venous thrombosis

Chest Pain

Chest pain is a patient complaint for which the causes range from postgastric-procedure "gas" pain to angina pectoris and myocardial infarction. Attempting to calmly differentiate the causes of chest pain can help you to focus on appropriate interventions and necessary communication with appropriate health care personnel.

- Ask the patient what makes the pain better or worse.
  - Pain that is relieved by sublingual nitroglycerin or stopping the activity that triggered the pain may suggest that the pain is cardiac in nature.
- Ask the patient to describe the pain symptoms.
  - Pain that is described as squeezing, a tightness in the center of the chest, a feeling of a lump in the throat, or a heavy weight on the chest may be cardiac. The patient may describe the pain to you while pressing his or her clenched fist against the chest (pressure and constriction). This is termed the *Levine sign*. The patient may rate the pain as a "10" on a 0 to 10 scale—the worst pain ever experienced.
    - A woman may describe cardiac pain as more like heartburn, burning, "stomach upset," or indigestion (causing her to delay seeking treatment).
    - Women may break out in a cold sweat or feel extreme fatigue.

- Ask the patient whether the pain is radiating and to where.
  - Pain occurring in a small area in the chest is likely originating from the lungs.
  - Cardiac pain is not localized; if the pain radiates to several areas, it is most likely cardiac.
  - Pain that radiates to the neck, throat, lower jaw, teeth, upper extremities, or shoulder is most likely cardiac.
    - Arm, back, neck, and jaw pain is more common in women experiencing cardiac pain.
- Is the pain radiation occurring with other symptoms? Other cardiac symptoms include nausea, vomiting, sweating, feeling faint, shortness of breath, dizziness, palpitations, and fatigue.
- What is the pain severity on a 0 to 10 scale? Be aware that the severity of the pain is not necessarily related to the degree of ischemia. In women, pain may be absent.
- Does the pain occur in association with actions such as exercise or eating?
  - Chest pain that occurs with exercise/exertion is a symptom of angina.
  - Ischemic chest pain can also be caused by cold, stress, smoking, eating a large meal (may also be gastric disease), or engaging in sexual intercourse.
- How long does the pain last?
  - Cardiac pain usually occurs gradually and increases over time. Chest pain that occurs suddenly is usually associated with pneumothorax, aortic dissection, or pulmonary embolism.
  - Ischemic pain lasts for a few minutes, whereas pain from a myocardial infarction lasts longer.
  - Chest pain that lasts for several hours or over a period of days is probably not due to ischemia.

As is the case with many disease symptoms in the elderly, their presentation of chest pain is not typical. For example, the pain may be vague, nonspecific, and located in the abdomen or epigastric area. They may only complain of shortness of breath on exertion or rest, fatigue, feeling faint, or gastrointestinal complaints of nausea and anorexia.

Heart Failure

Heart failure is the inability of the heart to pump a sufficient amount of blood to adequately meet the oxygen demands of the cells and tissues of the body. It is the result of a variety of cardiac conditions, including chronic hypertension, valve disease, and coronary artery disease. The effects of either right- or left-sided ventricular failure are similar and therefore cannot be used to differentiate the types. Signs and symptoms of heart failure include:

- Pale, cyanotic skin and nail beds
- Dependent edema
- Decreased activity tolerance and ability to perform ADL
- Altered mental status
- Tachycardia, S3 heart sound, heart murmurs, and increased jugular vein distention
- Lightheadedness, dizziness, and confusion
- Chest pain along with shortness of breath
- Shortness of breath that occurs at night (paroxysmal nocturnal dyspnea)
- Dyspnea on exertion
- Bilateral crackles that do not clear with cough. Rhonchi may also be present
- Cough when lying supine
- Cough with exertion
- Orthopnea
- Nausea, possible vomiting, and anorexia, but weight gain due to fluid accumulation
- Ascites
- Decreased urinary output during the day followed by nocturia
- Blood pressure may be high or low depending on severity of heart failure

Nursing interventions include:

- Auscultate apical pulse, noting dysrhythmias and heart sounds
- Monitor blood pressure, which may be elevated in early heart failure, later developing hypotension

- Palpate bilateral pulses, which may be bounding then weak
- Monitor urine output; it may decrease during the day and increase at night
- Monitor mental status, noting onset of lethargy, confusion, or disorientation (hypoxemia or altered electrolyte levels)
- Encourage bed rest in semi-Fowler's position
- Elevate legs, encourage active/passive exercises
- Administer medications as ordered
- Monitor and report electrolytes—fluid shifts can affect their levels; monitor and report other ordered lab work (possibly kidney and liver function)
- Monitor and report electrocardiogram (EKG)/heart monitor results
- Note and report adventitious breath sounds
- Note and report presence of or increasing edema
- Note and report upper abdominal pain (can indicate liver engorgement)
- Provide supplemental oxygen as needed
- Monitor skin integrity

Angina Pectoris

Angina pectoris is defined as paroxysmal, severe constricting chest pain or pressure in the anterior of the chest that is caused by myocardial ischemia or lack of oxygen to the cells of the heart. The pain often radiates to one or both shoulders, neck, or jaw. It is caused by exertion, exposure to cold, eating a heavy meal, or emotional stress. There are five types of angina:

- Stable—pain that occurs with exertion and that is relieved by rest and lasts less than 15 minutes.
- Unstable—pain can occur with rest and exertion. It is longer lasting, occurs more frequently, and is not relieved by rest or nitroglycerin.

- Intractable—severe, incapacitating pain
- Variant (variable)—caused by coronary artery spasms, the pain occurs at rest
- Silent ischemia—patient reports no signs or symptoms; however, there are EKG changes suggestive of ischemia during stress testing.

Signs and symptoms of angina pectoris include:

- Pain ranging from mild (indigestion) to "heavy feeling" to agonizing
- Severe apprehension and feeling of "impending doom"
- Pain is often located behind the sternum (retrosternal)
- Pain radiates to neck, jaw, shoulders, and inner aspect of the upper arms (left more than right)
  - Pain down both arms is typical in the elderly patient
  - Women may have pain between the shoulder blades or back or a dull backache
- Patient describes chest tightness as ranging from choking to strangling, with a viselike quality
  - Note that diabetics may not report this type of pain due to neuropathy.
- Arms, wrists, and hands may be reported to feel weak or numb
- Shortness of breath
  - Dyspnea may be the only symptom in the elderly patient
- Pallor
- Diaphoresis
- Nausea/vomiting
- Lightheadedness
- Severe pain may decrease the heart rate and blood pressure

Your *immediate* nursing interventions include the following. Please note that you will also be preparing the patient for transport to the coronary care unit.

- Place patient on bed rest in semi-Fowler's position
- Question the patient to ascertain whether this pain is the same/different than pain he or she has experienced in the

past. A difference may indicate worsening disease or a different cause than in the past.

- Monitor vital signs at least every 5 minutes. Patients experiencing angina may develop arrhythmias, tachycardia, and decreased blood pressure.
- Follow facility policy for obtaining and reporting the results of a 12-lead EKG.
- Provide supplemental oxygen of at least 2 liters per minute via nasal cannula. Monitor the oxygen saturation levels. Monitor for respiratory distress.
- Administer antianginal medication as ordered. Monitor the response of the pain to the medication. Follow facility guidelines for administration and patient assessment during medication administration.
- Administer other ordered medications as per facility policy.

Myocardial Infarction

When an area of the myocardium is destroyed due to reduced blood flow, it is termed a *myocardial infarction* (MI). MIs may be caused by occlusion of the coronary artery by a thrombus, constricting of the coronary artery due to vasospasm, decreased blood supply due to trauma or low blood pressure, or rapid heart rate such as that which occurs when ingesting cocaine. MIs are described by their type (i.e., segment elevation), location of the injury in the heart (i.e., anterior wall, lateral wall, and so on), and the current point of time in the process (i.e., acute, old, and evolving).

Signs and symptoms include:

- Chest pain, palpitations
- Possibly increased jugular venous distention (if MI caused by heart failure)
- Elevated blood pressure
- EKG changes showing tachycardia, bradycardia, or dysrhythmias

- Shortness of breath, dyspnea, tachypnea
- Cyanosis of the nail beds, lips, and mucous membranes; mottling of the skin
- Crackles in the lungs if the MI has caused pulmonary congestion
- Nausea/vomiting
- Skin is cold, clammy, diaphoretic, and pale
- Anxiety, restlessness, lightheadedness
- Feeling of impending doom, or the opposite—denial

Nursing interventions for the patient experiencing a heart attack include the following. Please note that you will also be preparing the patient for transport to the coronary care unit:

- Provide relief of chest pain following facility-approved medication protocols.
- Provide supplemental oxygen, usually 2 to 4 liters per minute via nasal cannula.
- Monitor oxygen saturation levels and maintain at 96% to 100%.
- Monitor vital signs frequently.
- Place patient on bed rest in semi-Fowler's position.
- Establish or maintain intravenous line access.
- Obtain and report EKG as per facility policy.
- Obtain and report ordered lab work, which may include cardiac enzymes, electrolyte levels, and arterial blood gases.
- Attempt to decrease anxiety.

Obtaining an EKG

Know your facility's guidelines for nursing staff obtaining an EKG. In many facilities, it is a nursing intervention for the nurse to obtain the EKG and provide the results for the MD. Figure 5.1 shows a guide to EKG lead placement.

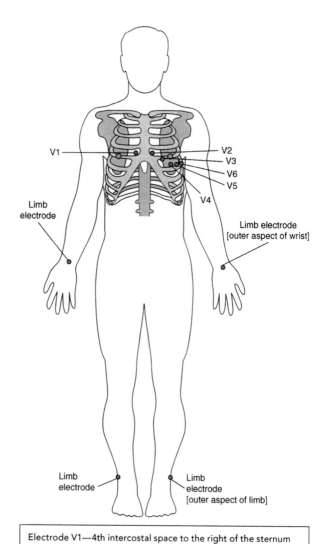

Electrode V1—4th intercostal space to the right of the sternum
Electrode V2—4th intercostal space to the left of the sternum
Electrode V3—midway between V2 and V4
Electrode V4—5th intercostal space at the midclavicular line
Electrode V5—anterior axillary line at the same level as V4
Electrode V6—midaxillary line at the same level as V4 and V5
Electrode RL—anywhere above the ankle and below the torso
Electrode RA—anywhere between the shoulder and the elbow
Electrode LL—anywhere above the ankle and below the torso
Electrode LA—anywhere between the shoulder and elbow

FIGURE 5.1   EKG lead placement.

The Partnership for Patients (http://partnershipforpatients .cms.gov) has identified the prevention of venous thromboembolism (VTE) as 1 of the 10 core patient safety areas in hospitalized patients. A VTE is a blood clot that forms within a vein. VTE is a deep vein thrombosis (DVT) that can break off and cause a pulmonary embolism (see Chapter 6). The terms DVT, VTE, and thrombophlebitis are oftentimes used interchangeably. Your assessments should include:

- Inspecting the patient's skin, noting color and temperature change and edema
- Noting and documenting the circumference of both ankles and calves and comparing them
- Noting redness, inflammation, or pain that is progressive from the lower extremities (for example, redness of the lower calf that is extending upward)
- Noting any prominent, superficial veins
- Assessing capillary refill
- Noting and reporting patient complaints of a limb feeling heavy or painful or that the patient may not be able to move the extremity as previously

====================================== *FAST FACTS in a NUTSHELL*

It is estimated that 1 in 100 hospitalized patients dies of pulmonary embolism, half of which were preventable.

Patients at risk for VTE include:

- Those who have suffered a traumatic injury to the lower legs
- Postoperative patients, especially orthopedic patients (legs, knees, and hips) and those who have had surgery lasting longer than 30 minutes
- Any patient with a venous catheter in place, including central lines and dialysis access

- Those patients who are obese
- Those with a history of cancer, especially in the pelvis
- Those with a history of DVT or pulmonary embolism
- Those on bed rest or who are immobile due to paralysis, spinal cord injury, or casting
- Those with varicose veins (and those who have undergone venous stripping)
- Those with a history of cardiac disorders, including history of MI and heart failure
- Patients with a history of stroke, nephritic syndrome, thrombocytosis, lupus, infections, and various diseases that alter their coagulation ability

A nurse's ability to recognize DVT is difficult because the signs are often vague and nonspecific. Common but ambiguous signs and symptoms of DVT include:

- Edema and swelling of an extremity (measure and compare both extremities)
- If both extremities are swollen, the affected extremity may be warmer than the unaffected and the superficial veins more prominent.
- Tenderness is a later sign, elicited by gentle palpation of the affected extremity.
- Pain in the calf when the foot is dorsiflexed (Homans' sign) is not specific for DVT. This pain can be caused by many conditions.

FAST FACTS in a NUTSHELL

Careful assessment and comprehensive interventions with at-risk patients may help to prevent a fatal embolism. In many cases the first symptom of a DVT was the pulmonary embolus.

The agreed method of prevention of VTE is aimed at either increasing venous blood flow to prevent clot formation (mechanical) or medication to slow blood coagulation (chemical). Nursing interventions to prevent VTE include:

- Early mobilization of a surgical patient, including short, frequent walks. If the patient is immobile, then perform passive range of motion of the lower extremities.
- If the patient is able, allow him or her to perform active range of motion of the lower extremities. This includes flexion/extension and rotation of the feet.
- Apply, as ordered, graded compression stockings and ensure that they fit properly; increased pressure at the ankle and decreasing toward the calf or above the knee
- Apply, as ordered, intermittent pneumatic leg compression. Follow facility guidelines for application times and duration.
- Teach the patient to avoid crossing his or her legs or to sit with legs dangling.
- Do not rub or massage the affected extremity. This can dislodge the thrombus. Teach the patient to do the same.
- Encourage postoperative deep-breathing exercises.
- Increase (if medically tolerated) daily fluid intake. Dehydration causes a decrease in blood viscosity and can increase the risk of clots.
- Follow MD orders for application of warm compresses. These can be contraindicated if your patient has arterial insufficiency.
- Administer anticoagulants as ordered and as per facility policy.
- Monitor necessary lab work, such as prothrombin time, partial thromboplastin time, and international normalized ratio, and promptly report findings.

6

Common Respiratory Conditions and Emergencies

Patients with chronic, long-standing respiratory disease are often admitted to the medical–surgical unit. You learn to be prepared to care for these patients, as the course of disease exacerbation and recovery is often repeated many times over and you see the same patients on many admissions. Other patients develop acute respiratory distress, and your assessment skills and communication with health care professionals are vitally important to saving their lives.

After reading this chapter, the reader will be able to:

1. List steps of a focused respiratory assessment
2. List signs and symptoms of chronic obstructive pulmonary disease
3. List signs and symptoms of pneumonia
4. Describe a "VAP bundle" and how it can eliminate ventilator-associated pneumonia (VAP) infection
5. Describe how to prevent atelectasis

RESPIRATORY ASSESSMENT BACKGROUND

While you engage your patient in conversation, you are assessing his or her breathing pattern, color, ease in speaking, position (i.e., leaning forward to breathe), cough, ease of ambulation, and orientation. Your patient may be admitted to your unit with a respiratory condition, but a respiratory emergency could develop within moments for any patient and you will need to assess and intervene quickly.

You should perform a more focused respiratory assessment if the patient experiences:

- Shortness of breath (a deviation from baseline)
- Restlessness and anxiety
- Cyanosis
- Abnormal breath sounds
- Rapid breathing/slow breathing (tachypnea or bradypnea)
- Leaning forward to breathe (tripod position)
- Difficulty speaking
- Retractions or using the accessory muscles to breathe
- Nasal flaring
- Pursed lip breathing
- Cough that becomes productive (sputum type, color, consistency is important to note)

A FOCUSED RESPIRATORY ASSESSMENT

On encountering any patient that you suspect may be experiencing a respiratory issue, you should immediately perform a focused assessment. All of the assessment techniques are used when examining the patient in respiratory distress, including inspection, palpation, auscultation, and percussion. Compare all findings to baseline and note any change. Be aware of the patient's previous respiratory health history. Included in this assessment should be a set of vital signs, including pulse oximetry. Note the rate and character of the respirations and pulse. Include a mental status check and note the patient's skin color and other objective changes.

- If there is dyspnea (shortness of breath), note the onset and contributing factors—was the onset sudden or gradual, are other symptoms present, what position was the patient in (supine, upright) when the dyspnea began?
- Assess breath sounds, noting adventitious breath sounds such as wheezing, rhonchi, crackles, or areas of decreased or absent breath sounds.

═══════════════════════════ *FAST FACTS in a NUTSHELL*

Turn and position the patient in order to auscultate all lung fields for ALL patients. Atelectasis or fluid in the lungs may be missed if all fields are not auscultated.

- Note respiratory rate and effort.
- Note presence and location of cyanosis. Central cyanosis (lips, earlobes) indicates advanced hypoxia.
- Note presence of anxiety or distress (due to air hunger/hypoxia).
- Monitor level of consciousness, noting change or decrease in sensorium.
- If there is cough, describe the type (dry, productive, persistent, hacking, or severe).
- If there is sputum, note the amount, color, and consistency.
- With cough, note the time of onset.
- Note breathing patterns.
  - Bradypnea—less than 10 breaths per minute, slow breathing, regular pattern—could indicate brain injury.
  - Tachypnea—more than 24 breaths per minute, rapid breathing, regular pattern—could indicate pneumonia, pulmonary edema.
  - Hypoventilation—irregular, shallow breathing
  - Hyperpnea—increase in depth of respiration
  - Hyperventilation—increase in depth and rate of respiration
  - Kussmaul's respiration—hyperventilation seen in diabetic ketoacidosis.

- Apnea—periods of absence of breathing
- Cheyne–Stokes—alternating periods of apnea and deep breathing; apneic periods may last for 5 to 30 seconds. Deep respirations become shallow. Document timing of both. Seen at the end of life, with heart failure, and in damage by trauma or tumor to the respiratory center of the brain.
- Biot's (cluster) irregular breathing with varying rate and depth—could indicate lesions in the brain stem.

- Note any medications that are prescribed and their side and adverse affects. These may contribute to respiratory symptoms (i.e., the dry cough caused by angiotensin-converting enzyme inhibitors).
- Note neck vein distention.
- Note the presence of peripheral edema.
- Note patient complaint of chest pain. Describe the quality, intensity, and radiation of the pain.
- Chest pain can be associated with either cardiac or respiratory disorders.
  - Pain that is respiratory in origin can be described as sharp, dull, intermittent, aching, or stabbing.
  - Pain can occur with inspiration or expiration.
  - Pain is usually located where pathology exists.
- Palpate the area of the pain, noting areas of tenderness, fremitus, lesions, masses
- Is the patient able to speak without losing his breath or having to stop to take a breath? Does the patient use pursed-lip breathing or have prolonged expirations?
- Percuss appropriate areas of the chest to determine presence of air, fluid, or masses.

FAST FACTS in a NUTSHELL

Auscultation of lung fields, current mental status, and measurement of pulse oximetry together determine the patient's respiratory status.

COMMON RESPIRATORY DISORDERS SEEN ON THE MEDICAL–SURGICAL UNIT

- Chronic obstructive pulmonary disease (COPD)
- Pulmonary emboli
- Pneumonia
- Atelectasis

Chronic Obstructive Pulmonary Disease

COPD is an umbrella term used to describe any respiratory disease characterized by obstructed airflow, including emphysema and chronic bronchitis. The disease is progressive, with patients becoming symptomatic during their middle adult years and worsening as the patient grows older. As the patient is exposed to lung irritants (i.e., from smoking) the injury and repair process occurring in the lung tissues causes the airways to narrow and scars to form. In emphysema, airway obstruction is caused by parenchymal destruction.

Signs and symptoms of COPD include:

- Fatigue, inability to sleep
- Persistent cough with sputum production; sputum is gray, white, or yellow and may be copious.
- Inability to perform activities of daily living (ADL), so patient may have poor hygiene
- Weight loss, poor appetite, or inability to eat due to dyspnea

═══════════════════════════*FAST FACTS in a NUTSHELL*

The classic signs of COPD include chronic cough, sputum production, and dyspnea on exertion.

- Dependent edema
- Tachycardia, dysrhythmias, or elevated blood pressure (BP)
- Pale skin and mucous membranes; cyanosis of the lips and nail beds
- Faint breath sounds with expiratory wheezing (emphysema); scattered crackles (bronchitis)
- Percussion of the chest wall reveals hyperresonance (emphysema) or dullness over areas of fluid or mucus
- Difficulty speaking due to breathlessness
- Rapid, shallow breathing; prolonged expiratory phase with pursed-lip breathing
- Use of accessory muscles in breathing, nasal flaring
- Dyspnea at rest and distended neck veins in advanced stages of disease

  Nursing interventions include:

- Elevate the head of the bed, or have the patient lean on an overbed table or assume the "tripod" position in order to promote oxygenation.
- Provide oxygen therapy as necessary.
- Increase fluid intake as tolerated.
- Administer medications as ordered (bronchodilators, inhalers, nebulizer treatments, anti-inflammatories, antimicrobials, or cough suppressants).
- Monitor and report abnormal test results.
- Suction patient as needed, noting amount, color, and consistency of sputum.
- Monitor vital signs, including cardiac rhythm, pulse oximetry and level of consciousness. Expect the pulse oximetry to be low. Oxygen therapy will not make it "normal." Monitor mental status and patient statements to determine whether oxygenation is adequate.
- Provide a quiet environment and promote rest.
- Monitor food intake and assist with feeding.
- Provide frequent oral care.
- Teach pulmonary hygiene.
- Teach pursed-lip-breathing technique, diaphragmatic breathing.

A pulmonary embolism (PE) is a sudden blockage of a pulmonary artery by a thrombus or clot that originated in the venous system (deep vein thrombosis [DVT]) or from the right side of the heart. PEs are a common disorder and are often associated with orthopedic surgery, trauma, age over 50 years, heart failure, and patients with prolonged immobility.

═══════════════════════════════════FAST FACTS in a NUTSHELL

Always suspect PE with high-risk patients who develop sudden, severe dyspnea and tachycardia.

Symptoms develop rapidly, with dyspnea, severe respiratory distress/failure, and tachypnea being the most common. Other symptoms include:

- Sudden chest pain that is worse with cough
- Anxiety (fear of impending doom)
- Fever
- Tachycardia
- Cough
- Diaphoresis
- Hemoptysis (coughing up blood)
- Syncope
- Jugular venous distention

═══════════════════════════════════FAST FACTS in a NUTSHELL

Death can occur within 1 hour of onset of PE symptoms. Assessment must be accurate and quick.

Nursing interventions include:

- Provide supplemental oxygen via nasal cannula immediately.

- Insert or maintain intravenous line access.
- Auscultate the lungs and note areas of decreased or absent breath sounds.
- Observe for generalized cyanosis.
- Monitor vital signs, noting changes in cardiac rhythm, tachycardia, dysrhythmias, tachypnea, and blood pressure changes.
- Monitor level of consciousness and changes in mentation.
- Elevate the head of the bed to promote oxygenation.
- Monitor pulse oximetry.
- Place heart monitor in place to assess for onset of dysrhythmia.
- Administer medications as ordered.
- Insert indwelling urinary catheter as ordered (to monitor urine output).
- Prepare patient for diagnostic testing, such as perfusion scans, computed tomography scans, pulmonary angiography and laboratory work.
- Prepare patient for transport to intensive care.
- Initiate emergency care for respiratory arrest if necessary.

Pneumonia

Pneumonia is an inflammation of the lung parenchyma. It can be caused by inhaled irritants, bacteria (90%), viruses, fungi, or aspiration. Community-acquired pneumonia is caused by gram-negative organisms. It is a major cause of death in the elderly. Health care–acquired or nosocomial pneumonia begins 48 hours after admission to a hospital. It accounts for 15% of all hospital-acquired infections. Signs and symptoms of pneumonia vary and depend on the organism causing the infection.

If caused by a streptococcal organism: sudden onset of chills, high fever, chest pain aggravated by breathing and coughing, tachypnea, shortness of breath, and rapid bounding pulse. Other pneumonia symptoms include:

- Fatigue, weakness
- Tachycardia
- Flushed skin, pallor, or central cyanosis
- Loss of appetite, nausea/vomiting

- Dry skin, poor skin turgor
- Headache
- Changes in mental status due to hypoxia
- Chest pain aggravated by cough
- Progressive dyspnea
- Cough—dry and hacking progressing to productive
- Sputum may be scanty or copious (pink, rusty, green, yellow, or white)
- On auscultation—pleural friction rub, dullness, fremitus
- Diminished or absent breath sounds
- Pale or cyanotic lips and nail beds
- Chills and fever

Nursing interventions include:

- Monitor depth and rate of respirations
- Watch for signs of impending respiratory failure
- Auscultate lung fields, noting adventitious sounds, or diminished/absent of breath sounds
- Elevate head of bed
- Suction as needed
- Encourage fluids if not contraindicated to thin secretions
- Administer medications as ordered, including nebulizer treatments, analgesics, expectorants, and antibiotics
- Provide supplemental oxygen
- Monitor lab work and other ordered tests and report abnormalities
- Encourage deep breathing and use of incentive spirometer

In order to prevent the onset of pneumonia:

- Use standard precautions
- Turn and position the patient frequently
- Promote coughing and deep-breathing exercises
- Suction as needed, provide frequent oral hygiene
- Monitor enteral feedings
- Obtain speech therapy consultation on those patients with swallowing difficulties.
- Elevate the head of the bed for patients with enteral feedings and in others not medically contraindicated.
- Only use clean (or sterile) respiratory equipment and supplies and follow strict hand hygiene practices.

Prevention of VAP

VAP is a health care–acquired infection in patients with endotracheal intubation on ventilators. It is the leading cause of death among health care–associated infections. The high morbidity and mortality of the ventilated patient from several factors, including VAP, led the Institute for Healthcare Improvement to develop the "Ventilator Bundle," five elements of care for the ventilated patient. Two of the elements are not related to the respiratory system, but through continued use in various health care settings, it was found that by following the bundle VAP was either dramatically reduced or eliminated altogether.

The VAP bundle elements are:

- Elevating the head of the bed between 30 and 45 degrees (if medically appropriate)
- Follow facility protocol when providing breaks in sedation and a daily assessment of the readiness to extubate the patient.
- Administer medication to prevent peptic ulcer.
- Follow facility guidelines in preventing DVTs.
- Follow facility protocol on oral care of the patient. Dental plaque biofilms are a reservoir for respiratory pathogens.

Atelectasis

Atelectasis is a reduction or absence of air in part or all of a lung—a dead space. It may be acute or chronic. It can occur in small areas not detectable on chest x-ray to loss of overall lung volume. Acute atelectasis is the most common, occurring in postoperative patients or in those patients who are immobile for long periods. When a patient does not take deep breaths either due to postoperative pain or immobility, respiratory secretions and mucous plugs obstruct airflow, causing atelectasis.

Signs and symptoms of atelectasis are subtle and include:

- Cough
- Sputum production

- Low-grade fever (may be caused by infection or inflammation not associated with the airway obstruction)
- Respiratory distress, if the atelectasis involves large portions of the lung
- Dyspnea
- Tachycardia, tachypnea
- Pleural pain
- Central cyanosis (late sign of hypoxia)
- Difficulty breathing when lying flat
- Anxiety

Nursing interventions to prevent atelectasis in the alert patient include:

- Get the patient out of bed as soon as possible after surgery from chair to ambulation.
- Frequently turn and position the immobilized patient—supine to upright.
- Implement deep-breathing and coughing exercises/use of incentive spirometer at least every 2 hours.
- Administer pain medication as needed so that patient does not avoid taking deep breaths due to pain; however, avoid respiratory depression.
- Assist in respiratory therapy as needed.
- Suction as needed.

If the patient is not able to perform coughing and deep breathing or if you are unable to mobilize the patient, other methods must be used. This can include positive end-expiratory pressure or continuous positive airway pressure.

METHODS OF OXYGEN DELIVERY

- **Nasal cannula**—Used for oxygen delivery of up to 6 liters per minute. The percentage of inspired oxygen ranges from 24% to 44%. The nasal mucosa can become dry and irritated if the oxygen is not humidified. Be aware of the potential for skin breakdown above the ears.

- **Simple face mask**—Used for short-term oxygen delivery of 5 to 8 liters per minute. Percentage of inspired oxygen ranges from 30% to 60%. This type of mask is contraindicated in patients with carbon dioxide retention because it can become worse.
- **Nonrebreather face mask**—(a mask with reservoir bag) delivers 60% to 90% oxygen with a flow rate of 6 to 10 liters per minute. The reservoir mask must be inflated throughout use to ensure that the patient is not inhaling exhaled carbon dioxide.
- **Venturi mask**—Delivers oxygen concentrations of 24% to 60% with flow rates between 4 and 12 liters per minute. The amount of oxygen can be specifically delivered. Humidified oxygen is delivered, which prevents the mucous membranes from drying. Be aware, however, that the humidified oxygen can irritate the patient's skin. Ensure that the mask fits properly or the amount of oxygen delivered will decrease.

The normal range of oxygen saturation is from 95% to 100%. If you have a reading of less than 90%, check for the following:

- Verify that the machine is charged.
- Do not take the low oxygen saturation reading in isolation. Monitor and observe the patient for other signs of decreased oxygenation, such as restlessness, tachycardia, cyanosis and anxiety.
- Does the patient have oxygen in place? If so, verify that it is infusing at the ordered rate and that the patient is in the most optimal position for ventilation (i.e., high Fowler's).

FAST FACTS in a NUTSHELL

Nurses suction patients in response to objective symptoms and oxygen saturation results. These should be documented. However, always assess and document oxygen saturation results *after* suctioning the patient. Was your intervention effective?

7

The Treatment of Common Gastrointestinal Conditions

As with many body systems, rapid assessment of patients with gastrointestinal (GI) issues is very important in order to avoid morbidity and death. GI emergencies can occur in patients with and without a previous GI diagnosis. Nasogastric tubes (NGTs) are common patient care equipment on a medical–surgical unit, but correctly caring for the patient using an NGT and the equipment itself is often overlooked. The information in this chapter provides information to assist you with effective care and monitoring of patients with GI conditions.

After reading this chapter, the reader will be able to:

1. List signs and symptoms of GI bleed
2. List signs and symptoms of a bowel obstruction
3. List the type of NGTs and their care
4. List how to care for the patient with an NGT

GASTROINTESTINAL ASSESSMENT BACKGROUND

Assessment of the GI system uses all four assessment techniques, including inspection, auscultation, palpation, and percussion. Remember that deep palpation is the last technique to be used, as it can lead to discomfort, pain, or the creation of bowel sounds that are inaccurate.

A FOCUSED GASTROINTESTINAL ASSESSMENT

Be familiar with the patient's medical and past history and be aware of any GI surgeries or procedures that the patient has had. Be aware of medications the patient is currently taking. Familiarize yourself with current lab work results that reflect the patient's nutritional and hydration status (metabolic panel, complete blood count, liver studies, iron, and triglycerides). Note any changes in weight and appetite. Document changes in bowel habits or character, food intolerances, history of vomiting, constipation and/or diarrhea, and how long these have occurred. Document any medications, including over-the-counter and herbal substances.

The most common symptom of a GI disorder is a complaint of indigestion. Be sure that you understand what the patient means by indigestion by questioning him or her for clarification.

- Does the patient mean she or he has heartburn or pain after eating?
- Does she or he have a feeling of bloating or fullness after eating?
- Also clarify whether a particular food causes the indigestion, such as fatty or spicy food or raw vegetables.
- Pain is a major symptom of GI disorder and it provides clues as to the cause. Note the pain's:
  - Location
  - Radiation
  - Duration
  - Frequency

- What brings on the pain and what relieves it (i.e., food, antacid, activity, rest, bowel movement)?
- Note nonverbal signs of pain, such as guarding.
- Note any complaint of excessive gas or flatulence, because it can be a symptom of gallbladder disease, allergy, or food intolerance.
- Inspect the bowel, noting distention or scars from previous surgeries.
- Auscultate the bowel and note the quality of bowel sounds.

═══════════════════════════════════*FAST FACTS in a NUTSHELL*

Normal bowel sounds occur every 5 to 15 seconds, lasting several seconds each. You must listen in each quadrant for at least 5 minutes to determine whether sounds are absent or hypoactive (less than 5 per minute), which can indicate ileus. Paradoxically, 35 bowel sounds or more per minute (hyperactivity) can indicate obstruction or inflammation. Report slowed, absent, or hyperactive bowel sounds.

- Percuss the abdomen in all quadrants to detect the presence of fluid, air, or masses. Do not percuss or palpate the abdomen if you suspect the patient has an aneurysm.
- Palpate the abdomen starting away from any areas that are painful and moving toward the painful area, using light palpation that progresses to deep. Note areas that illicit guarding or rigidity. Note any areas of pain or tenderness.

COMMON GASTROINTESTINAL CONDITIONS SEEN ON THE MEDICAL–SURGICAL UNIT

- GI bleed
- Small bowel obstruction
- Large bowel obstruction
- GI intubation

Gastrointestinal Bleed

GI bleeds can be caused by a variety of issues, including bleeding duodenal ulcer (most common), gastric ulcers, gastritis, severe bouts of vomiting, and stress ulcers. Less-common causes are esophagitis, gastric cancer, esophageal varices, hiatal hernia, hemophilia, and leukemia. Patients are usually directly admitted through the emergency room to the critical care unit when the bleed is severe. However, GI bleeds can develop in patients on the medical–surgical unit and patients are admitted there postoperatively.

Signs and symptoms of a GI bleed include:

- Patient complains of weakness, dizziness, or feeling tired.
- Vital sign assessment may reveal the following symptoms due to low circulating blood volume and decreased hemoglobin. Compare all vital signs to baseline.
  - Tachycardia and possible dysrhythmias
  - Tachypnea
  - Hyperventilation
  - Hypotension
  - Weak, thread pulse
  - Slow capillary refill
  - Cyanosis or pallor (may or may not be present if blood loss is low)
- Diaphoresis may be present due to pain or impending shock from blood loss
- Patient may state he or she is having heart palpitations
- Change in bowel characteristics (diarrhea, dark, bloody, tarry, bright red, or foul smelling). Constipation may be present, especially if the patient has been taking antacids or antidiarrheals due to the changes in the stool. Stool that is bright red (frank blood) or maroon is an indication of a rapid upper GI bleed.
- Anorexia, nausea, vomiting; the characteristics of the vomitus or nasogastric drainage can assist you in determining the source of the blood.
  - Presence of bright red blood can indicate arterial bleeding.

- Presence of dark red blood may be old blood or venous blood, such as from varices.
- Stool that is coffee ground-like in appearance may mean that there is an ooze of blood. The blood has been partially digested.
- The presence of undigested food may indicate an obstruction.
- If vomiting is projectile, it could indicate pyloric outlet obstruction.

- GI disturbances, such as burping, feeling of heartburn, or indigestion.
- Weight loss
- Signs of poor hydration, including concentrated urine, elevated specific gravity, or dry mucous membranes all due to loss of fluid.
- Altered mental status depending on how much circulating fluid has been lost. Level of consciousness may range from drowsiness to coma because of decreased oxygenation.
- Complaint of pain; the description and the location of the pain can assist you in determining the cause of the pain.
  - Sudden onset of excruciating pain may indicate perforation.
  - Discomfort following meals may indicate gastritis.
  - Left to midepigastric pain radiating to the back may indicate a gastric ulcer.
  - Pain accompanied with vomiting or pain relieved by antacids may indicate a gastric ulcer.
  - Localized right to midepigastric pain with a burning or gnawing feeling after a meal and relieved by food or antacid may indicate a duodenal ulcer.
  - Midepigastric pain with burning and regurgitation may indicate gastroesophageal reflux disease.
  - Absence of pain with bleeding may indicate esophageal varices or gastritis.

Nursing interventions for a GI bleed include:

- Monitor vital signs, noting changes in blood pressure and pulse, which indicate decreased blood volume.

- Monitor patient for signs and symptoms of shock and report immediately.
- Monitor intake and output (estimated from blood loss, vomitus, stools, and nasogastric suction) and any intravenous (IV) fluids received.
- Begin or maintain IV fluids.
- Monitor blood replacement therapy.
- Maintain patient on bed rest.
- Monitor for continued bleeding.
- Monitor for signs of disseminated intravascular coagulation, which can begin if there is an inadequate replacement of clotting factors. Signs and symptoms include: bleeding gums, nose bleed, appearance of bruises with minimal trauma, or oozing from past IV or intramuscular injection sites.
- Insert or maintain NGT
- Administer medications as ordered, which may include proton pump inhibitors, antiulcer agents, antacids, anticholinergics, vasoconstrictors, and antiemetics.
- Monitor and report lab values, such as hemoglobin, hematocrit, red blood cell count, and kidney function.
- Assist and/or prepare patient for diagnostic testing.

Bowel Obstruction

A bowel obstruction occurs when the normal flow of intestinal contents is impeded by one of three means.

- *Mechanical* obstruction occurs when the lumen of the intestinal wall becomes narrowed by tumors, adhesions, strictures, diverticulitis, ulcerative colitis, hernias, or abscesses. The most common causes are adhesions and hernias.
- *Functional* obstruction occurs when the intestinal wall muscles do not propel the intestinal contents along the length of the bowel because an area of it stops functioning for more than 72 hours. Causes include muscular dystrophy, trauma, hypokalemia, myocardial infarction,

diabetes mellitus, vascular insufficiency, or Parkinson's disease. It can also be a side effect of anesthesia, medication (diuretics and antihypertensives), or extensive bowel manipulation during surgery. An obstruction can occur in the small or large bowel.

FAST FACTS in a NUTSHELL

Functional or adynamic obstruction is the most common type of obstruction—another term for it is *paralytic ileus.*

- *Vascular* obstruction occurs if the blood supply to a part of the bowel is blocked by a blood clot or thrombus in the mesenteric artery.

Small bowel obstruction occurs when intestinal contents, fluid, and gas accumulate above an obstruction. Ninety percent of bowel obstructions are in the small bowel, at the ileum.

FAST FACTS in a NUTSHELL

Bowel obstruction has a high mortality rate if not recognized and treated within 24 hours.

Symptoms of obstruction occur when the intestine can no longer absorb nutrients so it retains fluid (7 to 8 liters), which increases gastric secretion production. The retained fluid and increased fluid production together cause distention, placing pressure on the intestinal blood circulation. This in turn can lead to eventual necrosis and/or perforation of the intestine. Signs and symptoms also depend on the location, length of the obstruction, available blood supply, and what is causing the obstruction.

- Crampy, wavelike, rhythmic colicky pain (initial symptoms, caused by peristalsis)

- Pain from the small intestine is felt in the upper abdomen and midabdomen. Pain originating in the colon (colonic) is felt in the lower abdomen.
- Tachycardia from hypovolemia and possible bowel ischemia
- High-pitched tinkling bowel sounds
- Patient does not pass stool or flatus.
- Patient passes mucus and blood.
- Progressive vomiting of stomach, intestinal contents, and bile until finally vomiting fecal matter.
- Signs and symptoms of dehydration
- Distended abdomen (the lower the obstruction, the more distended the abdomen); severe distention inhibits breathing, causing hypoxia
- Hypovolemic shock due to dehydration and loss of fluid volume (if the obstruction is complete and not surgically corrected)

Nursing interventions for bowel obstruction include:

- Insert and maintain NGT (incomplete bowel obstruction can very often be decompressed with an NGT and the patient monitored for worsening symptoms).
- Insert and maintain IV therapy.
- Monitor intake and output.
- Monitor for fluid imbalance.
- Monitor and report abnormal lab work, noting electrolytes lost due to vomiting; profound loss of fluid and electrolytes can lead to metabolic acidosis.
- Monitor bowel sounds (note absence or renewed presence).
- Assess for renewed passage of stool and flatus.
- Monitor and report worsening signs of obstruction (increased abdominal pain, increased NGT output, or worsening distention).
- Prepare patient for possible surgery if medical treatment fails to relieve the obstruction.

A large bowel obstruction occurs when intestinal contents, fluid, and gas accumulate below an obstruction. Cancerous tumors cause 80% of the obstructions of the large bowel, the most common area being the sigmoid colon. In comparison to a small bowel obstruction, signs and symptoms develop more slowly and can depend on the location of the obstruction. Signs and symptoms include:

- Constipation (may occur over many months with no other symptoms; may be present in an obstruction in the sigmoid or the rectum)
- Stool character changes and becomes thin due to passing by the obstruction prior to evacuation.
- Blood in the stool (occult blood) may become evident as iron-deficiency anemia.
- Weakness and fatigue
- Abdominal distention (later symptom)
- Patient may not vomit in the early stages because the ileo-cecal valve is preventing the regurgitation of intestinal contents; however, in late stages of the condition vomiting will occur because small bowel also becomes obstructed.
- Anorexia and weight loss (unable to take in nutrients)
- Crampy, lower abdominal pain

    Nursing interventions for large bowel obstruction include:

- Monitor the patient for worsening of obstruction.
- Administer IV fluids.
- Monitor and report abnormal lab work (i.e., electrolytes).
- Insert, monitor, and maintain NGT.
- Prepare the patient for surgery if the symptoms do not improve.

Gastrointestinal Intubation

Patients have gastric or duodenal tubes for a variety of reasons, but it is more common on a medical–surgical unit for patients to have these tubes for decompression and tube feeding.

- Decompression—to eliminate gas from the stomach and intestine in order to treat obstruction or postoperatively in GI surgery patients to remove gastric secretions

- Tube feeding or enteral nutrition—gives fluid and nutrients via a tube into the stomach or small intestine with poor oral intake or in those with difficulty swallowing

There are several different types of tubes and the most common are:

- Short tubes include Levin (single lumen) and Salem (double lumen) Sump (the most common) tubes, which extend into the stomach but not the bowel. Set to suction low intermittent (Levin tube) or low continuous (Salem Sump). A Salem Sump tube, known for its blue "pigtail" and tubing vents, is most often used for irrigation and withdrawal of stomach contents and is the tube usually associated with stomach decompression. Both can be used for short-term feeding but they are associated with a high risk of aspiration pneumonia.
- Medium tubes include Dobhoff tubes, which extend into the duodenum. They are used for short-term feeding and have a lower rate of aspiration pneumonia.
- Long-term enteral feeding tubes include gastrostomy (GT and G) tubes or jejunostomy (JT or J) tubes. They are placed surgically, and the most common are percutaneous endoscopic gastrostomy tubes.

NGT USER HINTS

- Do not use the blue "pigtail" lumen in a Salem Sump tube for feeding or irrigation. It will stop functioning. The "pigtail" equalizes the atmospheric air and suction and works to keep the tube from coming in contact with the stomach wall.

FAST FACTS in a NUTSHELL

Listen for the whistle from the "pigtail." It indicates that the main tube is functioning and not in contact with the stomach mucosa.

- Do not clamp the "pigtail."
- Insert an antireflux valve into the blue lumen to prevent backflow of stomach contents into the valve.
- Maintain the end of the tube with the "pigtail" above the waist. Falling below this point will allow for backflow of suctioned material.
- At the start of your shift, ensure that suction settings are correct and the pump or wall suction is functioning, and note the amount and character of the gastric output. Make sure all tubing connections are secure.
- If the tube has stopped functioning, first insufflate air ONLY through the "pigtail." This will move the tip of the tube away from the stomach wall. This should be sufficient to have suction begin again.
- Do not advance or pull back on the tubing without verifying placement via the facility-approved method.
- Irrigation may be necessary if the tube is blocked, despite efforts to re-establish suction. Follow facility guidelines for irrigation procedures and measurement of intake/output.
- Re-establish suction after irrigation by instilling 20 mL of air through the "pigtail."
- Setting the suction on a Levin tube higher than low will contribute to stomach mucosa erosion.

CARE OF PATIENTS WITH NGTs

- Remember that the tube constantly irritates the nasal mucosa and is very uncomfortable for the patient. Monitor the skin and mucus for breakdown. Lubricating the nares with a nonpetroleum-based product helps to prevent irritation.
- Anchor the tube to the patient's face as per facility guidelines, using the proper anchor device and changing as per guidelines in order to prevent irritation from a soiled anchor.
- The tube allows for the patient to breathe only through one nare. The patient will usually breathe through his or her mouth. Ensure that the patient receives frequent mouth care and lip balm to keep lips moist.

- It may be permissible for the patient to rinse his or her mouth with cool water; do not allow the patient to swallow.
- Turn and position the patient frequently to assist with emptying of the stomach contents.
- Stomach irrigant contains electrolytes and loss may lead to fluid volume deficit and metabolic alterations. Monitor lab work and report deficits.

8

Promoting Safety and Preventing Infection in Patients With Genitourinary Alterations

Urinary tract issues are common in the hospitalized patient—common, but they should not become a normal event for the patient. Focused nursing assessments and interventions can assist the patient in preventing infection. Health care–associated urinary tract infections (UTIs) can be deadly to the hospitalized patient, so every effort must be taken to prevent this complication. The elderly patient may suffer from a UTI, but not display common symptoms, so nurses must be aware of alternate signs of infection and act accordingly.

After reading this chapter, the reader will be able to:

1. List the symptoms of a UTI
2. List how to prevent a catheter-associated UTI (CAUTI)
3. List how to prevent a UTI
4. List risk factors for a urinary tract disorder
5. List factors to prevent transient incontinence in the hospitalized patient

GENITOURINARY ASSESSMENT BACKGROUND

During your comprehensive assessment, note any genitourinary risk factors. Keep in mind that an acute illness and being in the hospital increase the patient's risk of developing a urinary tract dysfunction.

A FOCUSED GENITOURINARY ASSESSMENT

When questioning a patient, be aware that he or she may be embarrassed to discuss urinary issues or personal hygiene habits. As always, your questions should be posed in nonmedical terms and be easy for the patient to understand. In a focused assessment, you should ascertain:

- General past medical information with health history (acute illness or UTIs)
- If there is incontinence, inquire as to when it began and its severity.
- Note complaints of nocturia, hematuria, hesitancy, urgency, or painful urination.
- If there is a complaint of pain, note the location and duration. Note whether it occurs with voiding. Note what relieves the pain.
- Note the presence of fever.
- Obtain a list of all medications, including over-the-counter and herbal remedies the patient is taking. Many types of medications can cause altered urinary tract symptoms.
- Note suprapubic distention, which may indicate urinary retention.
- Request urinalysis and urine culture (with sensitivity) if you suspect a UTI. Report abnormalities.

FAST FACTS in a NUTSHELL

While bathing the patient, observe the genitalia for abnormalities, such as irritation, redness, drainage, wounds, or lesions.

> The presence of pain, changes in voiding, changes in the character of the urine, and gastrointestinal symptoms are strongly indicative of a urinary tract issue that must be assessed.

RISK FACTORS FOR GENITOURINARY DISORDERS

Prior medical conditions can place a patient at risk of developing renal and urologic disorders. These include:

- Family history of renal disease
- Pregnancy and obstetrical surgery
- Advanced age
- History of childhood illness, such as "strep throat" or nephritic syndrome
- Immobilization
- Exposure to toxic chemicals
- Hypertension
- Spinal cord injury
- Benign prostatic hypertrophy
- Trauma from pelvic surgery
- Introduction of instrumentation into the urinary system, such as catheters or cystoscopy scopes
- Neurological disorders such as Parkinsonism, diabetic neuropathy, and multiple sclerosis (MS)

COMMON GENITOURINARY DISORDERS SEEN ON THE MEDICAL–SURGICAL UNIT

Some of the most common genitourinary issues that develop on a medical–surgical unit include the following:

- UTI
- CAUTI
- Urinary incontinence

Urinary Tract Infection

The bladder is a sterile environment, maintained due to the outflow of the urine, the presence of enzymes that help to prohibit bacterial growth, and the physical barrier of the urethra. When these mechanisms are overcome by bacteria, usually from fecal contamination, a UTI occurs. There are two types of UTIs, which are classified by their location and as complicated or uncomplicated. These types include:

- Lower UTIs (cystitis, prostatitis, urethritis)
- Upper UTIs (infections of the kidney)
- Uncomplicated lower or uncomplicated upper UTIs include community (not health care–associated) infections. These are the most common and the most familiar to the public.
- Complicated lower and upper UTIs include the health care–associated infections, and in those patients with previous abnormalities, these place them at higher risk.

FAST FACTS in a NUTSHELL

The diagnosis of a UTI is based on patient symptoms and urine culture results. Both must be considered together for a definitive diagnosis. Positive urine culture or symptoms alone do not confirm a diagnosis. The patient's bladder may be colonized with bacteria and show no signs of infection.

Risk factors for UTI include:

- Incomplete bladder emptying
- Obstructed urine flow due to strictures or abnormalities in the urinary tract
- Kidney stones
- Neurologic abnormalities
- Catheter insertion that introduces bacteria into the system
- Contributing medical conditions, such as diabetes, which increases glucose levels in the urine, creating a friendly environment for the growth of bacteria

- Pregnancy
- Any condition that does not allow complete emptying of the bladder
- Contaminating the urethra by improperly cleansing the perineum
- Avoiding the urge to urinate

Signs and symptoms of a UTI include the following; however, note that many patients, especially the elderly, may be positive for a UTI, but have no symptoms.

- Positive urine culture (follow facility guidelines for parameters)
- Fever
- Cloudy and/or dark amber urine
- Painful urination
- Burning on urination
- Frequency
- Nausea/vomiting
- Nocturia
- Incontinence
- Suprapubic pain/back pain
- Hematuria
- Urgency
- Complicated UTIs can develop in patients with indwelling catheters. Patients may be asymptomatic except for increased bacteria counts; however, sepsis with shock can also occur.

FAST FACTS in a NUTSHELL

In the elderly, symptoms of a UTI may include altered mentation, lethargy, new-onset incontinence, or low-grade fever without any signs of UTI.

Nursing interventions for the patient with a UTI include:

- Administering medication such as antispasmodics, analgesics, antipyretics, and antibiotics

- Encourage the patient to drink water (better than other fluids) to increase hydration and promote increased urine flow.
- Advise the patient to avoid eating or drinking urinary tract irritants, such as coffee, tomatoes, spices, alcohol, and citrus.
- Encourage the patient to empty his or her bladder every 2 to 3 hours to flush out the bacteria.
- Educate the patient to cleanse the perineum from front to back after bowel movements. Ensure that all staff performing hygiene for the patient clean the patient in the same way.

Urinary Incontinence

Incontinence, or the loss of ability to control urine, is a common but not normal occurrence in patients of any age. Symptoms of incontinence resemble other medical conditions and should be verified by testing. Symptoms include:

- Symptoms that resemble a UTI, such as pain on urination and frequency
- Inability to urinate
- Weakness in urine stream
- Leakage of urine during activities or leakage that began after surgery
- Loss of urine before getting to the restroom
- Frequent bladder infections

There are two types of urinary incontinence: transient and established. **Transient or acute urinary incontinence** occurs suddenly with normally reversible symptoms. Thirty-six percent of patients will develop this type of incontinence during a hospital admission. **Established or chronic incontinence may have a sudden or gradual onset.** Ten to 42% of patients may be living with this type of incontinence. Once a person is admitted with an acute illness, the disorder becomes more evident and difficult for them to deal with. Types of established incontinence include:

- Stress—occurs with increased intra-abdominal pressure, such as that caused by laughing, sneezing, coughing, and lifting heavy objects.
- Urge—associated with the inability to control the feeling of urgency. Other signs include frequency, nocturia, and incontinence at night. Older adults are more prone to this type of incontinence due to normal age-related changes in the bladder.
- Mixed—a combination of stress and urge incontinence with symptoms of both
- Overflow—caused by an overdistended bladder. Urinary retention, uncomfortable bladder fullness, leakage, hesitancy, and dribbling are related to bladder outlet obstruction. Patients with benign prostatic hyperplasia, MS, and diabetes may have this type of incontinence.
- Functional—caused by cognitive or physical impairments that prevent the patient from urinating as usual. This includes those with progressive dementia who are unable to "find" the bathroom in time or a patient who is acutely ill and confused by the hospital environment.

In order for transient incontinence to be reversed the causes must be identified and treated. Causes of transient incontinence include:

- Delirium, confusion, or depression
- Atrophic vaginitis
- Medication
- Psychological disorders that affect patients' motivation
- Restricted mobility or environmental barriers
- Fecal impaction/constipation
- Urethritis
- Infection (UTI)
- Decreased fluid intake
- Caffeine and smoking
- Malnutrition and obesity

Urinary incontinence can impact the patient's health, safety, and quality of life. Injuries can include falls (often with fracture) because the patient is attempting to overcome loss of independence and does not wait for assistance in transfer or ambulation. Exposure to urine can cause skin irritation, skin breakdown, and pressure ulcers. The use of indwelling catheters can cause urethral injury and UTIs (see section on CAUTI).

Nursing interventions for patients with incontinence include:

- Be aware of the side effects of the patient's medications. Medications that may contribute to incontinence include diuretics, anticholinergics, antipsychotics, antidepressants, sedatives, hypnotics, alpha adrenergic blockers, and calcium channel blockers.
- Attempt to eliminate physical barriers that may prohibit the patient from using the bathroom facilities.
- Assess the patient's safety when transferring and using the toilet. If necessary, request a physical/occupational therapy consult for assistance.
- If appropriate, institute a toileting program.
- Teach and encourage the patient to begin pelvic floor muscle exercises.
- Administer medications as ordered for control of incontinence.
- Allow the patient to remain independent but avoid injury by keeping call lights within reach (answer them promptly) and providing elevated toilets, bedside commodes, and urinals or bedpans.
- Provide time for the patient to void prior to bedtime, leaving the unit for testing, or rehabilitation sessions.
- Clear the patient's room of obstacles and clutter. Keep the path to the bathroom clear.
- Ensure adequate fluid intake, although limit fluid a few hours prior to bedtime.
- Promote skin integrity by applying skin barrier ointments.
- The use of diapers promotes UTIs. Change absorbent products promptly.

It has long been a practice of health care professionals to insert an indwelling urinary catheter as a way to control urinary incontinence. The use of indwelling catheters places the patient at risk for infection, urethral erosion, and death. One of the greatest risks is UTIs. According to the Institute for Healthcare Improvement (IHI), over 5 million catheters are placed annually. UTIs account for 40% of health care–associated infections in hospitalized patients, 80% of which were caused by indwelling catheters. Also according to the IHI, nearly half of the placed catheters were done so for inappropriate reasons. *Inappropriate* reasons for catheters include:

- Staff convenience in incontinent patients
- To obtain a urine sample in a patient who can void
- Postoperatively, unless otherwise indicated for appropriate patients

Appropriate reasons for use of indwelling catheters in hospitalized patients are limited but include:

- To promote comfort for the dying patient
- To promote healing in incontinent patients with Stage 3 or 4 pressure ulcers (or other wounds) of the sacral or perineal area
- Previously diagnosed (and documented) urinary outlet obstruction or retention
- Need for accurately measured urinary output
- Patients with unstable spine injuries or multiple traumatic injuries
- Perioperatively (remove in postanesthesia care unit if indicated, or within 24 hours if possible)

FAST FACTS in a NUTSHELL

If the patient does not meet the criteria for an indwelling catheter, be empowered and be a patient advocate. Suggest the use of an external catheter for your male patient, bladder scanning, and intermittent catheterization and/or bladder training for all.

CAUTIs can be prevented by using the following guidelines:

- Insert an indwelling catheter only when its use meets the previous conditions.
- Discontinue the catheter as soon as medically feasible.
- Insert the catheter using sterile technique, using the tube (French) with the smallest bore possible.
  - Wash the perineal area with soap and water immediately prior to catheter insertion.
  - Perform hand hygiene immediately before and after insertion or care of the catheter.
  - Open the sterile container; maintain sterility at all times.
  - Wear sterile gloves.

FAST FACTS in a NUTSHELL

Bring an extra pair of sterile gloves and extra catheter or insertion kit to the patient's room. This way, if you break sterility at any point, you do not have to leave the room for extra supplies and can remain with the patient.

- Organize supplies on the sterile field.
- Lubricate the catheter as appropriate for the gender of the patient.
- Apply sterile drape as appropriate for the gender of the patient.
- Place a sterile tray between patient's legs.

- Clean the urethral meatus. For a female, do not allow the labia to close because it recontaminates the area. In an uncircumcised male, if the foreskin does not remain retracted, repeat the cleaning procedure.
- Prior to inserting the catheter, grasp it close to the tip to maintain greater control of the tubing.
- If the catheter touches any area prior to direct insertion into the meatus, obtain another catheter as the original is contaminated.
- Securely anchor the catheter, allowing for movement of the thigh, as per facility policy. This will ensure that the catheter does not damage the urethra.
- Place the drainage bag lower than the bladder and instruct the patient on the importance of maintaining the bag in this position.
- Throughout the time the catheter is in place, cleanse it with facility-approved solution. Ensure that all performing hygiene for the patient cleanse from the body down the catheter toward the drainage bag. This will prohibit any bacteria from traveling up the catheter and into the urethra.

- Maintain the catheter based on facility guidelines, for instance, cleaning and duration of use and changing.
- Monitor the urine color, odor, and consistency. Note presence of sediment or cloudiness.
- Obtain urine samples using aseptic technique. Clean the port as per facility guidelines.

=== *FAST FACTS in a NUTSHELL*

Avoid obtaining urine samples from catheters that have been in place for long-term use. The sample will be contaminated. If appropriate, change the catheter and obtain a fresh urine sample.

- Promote the use of antibiotics for those patients who have symptomatic UTIs only.

- Maintain a closed drainage system. If the catheter disconnects or leaks, replace the entire catheter and drainage tubing.
- Empty the collection bag regularly with a clean container, one for each patient (label the container with the patient's name and room number and store as per facility guidelines).
- Routine bladder irrigation is *not* recommended. Do not irrigate a catheter without a specific order.

9

Promoting Healing, Preventing Altered Skin Integrity, and Preventing Wound Infection

The prevention and monitoring of wounds have always been one of the main responsibilities of the nurse. Technique for infection prevention in wound care cannot be forgotten, nor can techniques in preventing pressure ulcers. Unfortunately, health care institutions still have a high rate of acquired pressure ulcers and surgical site infections, so much so that the Institute for Healthcare Improvement (IHI) has developed guidelines for their prevention.

After reading this chapter, the reader will be able to:

1. List how to prevent a pressure ulcer
2. List the steps in assessing a surgical wound
3. List how to prevent an infection in a surgical site
4. List how to assess a wound
5. List how to assess a pressure ulcer

INTEGUMENTARY ASSESSMENT BACKGROUND

When performing a skin assessment, you will use the skills of not only inspection and palpation but your sense of smell as well. Skin assessments can be completed separately or when completing the overall physical assessment of the patient.

A FOCUSED INTEGUMENTARY ASSESSMENT

A focused skin assessment should be completed any time an alteration in skin integrity is found.

- Note the color of the lesion.
- Determine whether there is redness, pain, or swelling.
- Measure the size of the lesion using mm or cm (do not use common equivalents such as "dime size" or "quarter size," as they are less precise).
- Note the location of the lesion.
- Note whether there is drainage; note the color, odor, consistency, and amount.
- Determine whether there is a pattern to the lesion distribution, such as whether it follows a dermatome.

A focused wound assessment should be completed when the wound (continue from the above assessment if the lesion is a wound) is found before treatment and/or at regularly scheduled intervals, such as once a shift.

- Determine the cause of the injury. If caused while admitted, follow facility protocols for reporting and documenting.
- Determine whether there are foreign bodies in the wound.
- Measure the diameter and depth of the wound.
- If there is drainage, note the color, odor, consistency, and amount.
- Describe the wound bed and whether there is any necrotic or granulation tissue.
- Determine whether there is undermining and measure it if present.

- Measure and note whether there is erythema surrounding the wound.
- Assess skin surrounding the wound for redness or irritation.

A focused surgical site assessment should be completed postoperatively, during at least every shift and as needed.

- If the wound is covered by the original dressing, do not remove it unless ordered. Assess the wound only from the dressing and any drainage. Circle the amount of drainage directly on the dressing and write the date and time. This way you can determine whether further drainage occurs.
- If the patient is a fresh postop, don clean gloves and feel the sheet underneath the patient. If the wound is bleeding, it may not be evident on the dressing, but the blood will drain underneath the dressing and pool under the patient.

Once the original dressing is removed, note the following:

- Note whether the edges of the wounds are closing or approximated. There may be crusts of dried exudate along the wound edges—this is to be expected. A surgical wound should completely close within 7 to 10 days.
- Note whether there is any evidence of the wound separating or dehiscence.
- Note and document the number of staples or sutures present and whether they are intact. It is normal for the skin around the staples or sutures to be swollen for several days after surgery. If after 3 days the skin remains swollen, inform the physician, as this indicates the staples or sutures are too tight, which can lead to dehiscence.
- Gently palpate the wound edges, noting any pain, tenderness, or drainage (perform hand hygiene and wear gloves prior to palpation). Document whether the palpation causes drainage to exit the wound and whether there is extreme tenderness, as it could indicate infection.
- It is normal for the outer edges of a surgical wound to be red and inflamed for the first 2 to 3 days. This should resolve.

FAST FACTS in a NUTSHELL

Signs of infection in a surgical wound include swelling, drainage, and bright red inflammation.

- It is normal for bruising to appear near surgical wounds due to clotting underneath the tissues or the presence of a hematoma. The color will range from blue/purple and gradually fade to brown and yellow.
- There should be no drainage after 3 days; note and report its presence.
- If there is drainage, note the color, odor, consistency, and amount. Be aware that surgical wounds vary in the amount of drainage depending on where they are located; wounds with abscesses will have increased drainage.

FAST FACTS in a NUTSHELL

When documenting the amount of wound drainage, chart the amount of dressings used and how often the dressing was changed, thus an increase or decrease in either the amount of material or times changed will indicate the amount of drainage.

- Note the presence of drains near the surgical site and document their locations.
- Be careful when moving the patient or changing the dressing to avoid accidentally removing the drain.
- Document the amount of drains present, their location, and the character of the drainage (amount, color).
- Ensure that the drain is functioning; note drainage in the tubing and document at the end of the shift that the drains were intact and functioning.
- If there is an abnormal decrease or absence in the amount of drainage, notify the MD as the tubing or drain may be blocked.

- Assess and document that the suction device is in working order.
- If you suspect that the wound is infected, follow facility guidelines when obtaining a wound culture. Monitor the patient's temperature and report fever.
- If the surgical wound bleeds bright red excessive blood, obtain a set of vital signs, call the MD, and apply pressure to the wound.

COMMON INTEGUMENTARY DISORDERS SEEN ON THE MEDICAL–SURGICAL UNIT

The most common integumentary issues seen on a medical–surgical unit include the following:

- Pressure ulcers
- Surgical wounds
- Wounds

Pressure Ulcers

According to the 2007 National Pressure Ulcer Advisory Panel (NPUAP), the definition of a pressure ulcer is a localized injury to the skin and/or underlying tissue usually over a bony prominence, as a result of pressure or pressure in combination with shear. The most common sites of pressure ulcers are the sacrum and heels.

Staging of Pressure Ulcers

Facilities with a wound-care nurse or team allow them to stage pressure ulcers. In other facilities without such resources, RNs are taught and expected to stage wounds and document them. Be aware of who may stage pressure ulcers in your facility.

- **Stage I/nonblanchable erythema**—Skin is intact with noted warmth or coolness; tissue may feel firm, soft, or boggy and the patient may experience pain or itching at the site.

The ulcer has defined borders and is reddened in light-skinned people and red, blue, or purple in darker-skinned patients. Skin does not blanch when pressed. This stage is also an indicator of an "at-risk" patient.

- **Stage II/partial thickness**—The skin breaks. Noted to be an abrasion, blister (with serous or serosanguinous fluid), or shallow crater with a red–pink wound bed. No slough is present. Edema is present. Infection may develop at the site and drainage may be present. If bruising is present it represents a deep tissue injury.

- **Stage III/full thickness *skin* loss**—The ulcer extends into the subcutaneous tissue; however, bone, tendon, or muscle is not exposed. The depth of wound varies by the location on the body. For example, areas of the body with low fat content may have shallow ulcers, whereas areas of the body with high fat content can develop deeper wounds. Slough may be present but does not obscure the wound. Undermining and tunneling may also be present. Necrosis and drainage continue. Infection develops.

- **Stage IV/full thickness *tissue* loss**—A wound with the ulcer extending into the underlying muscle, tendon, fascia, joint and bone—all of which may be exposed. Slough and eschar may be present along with undermining and tunneling. As with Stage III wounds, the depth of wound varies by the location on the body. For example, areas of the body with low fat content may have shallow ulcers, whereas areas of the body with high fat content can develop deeper wounds. Osteomyelitis or osteitis can occur. Necrosis and infection continue.

- **Unstageable/full thickness skin or tissue loss, depth unknown**—In this full thickness wound the actual depth of the ulcer cannot be measured because the wound is completely obscured by slough and/or eschar lying within the wound bed. The slough and eschar are usually debrided and at that point the depth of the wound is determined (Stage III or Stage IV).

- **Suspected deep tissue injury (DTI), depth unknown—** According to the NPUAP, a suspected DTI is a purple or maroon localized area of discolored intact skin or blood-filled blister caused by damage of underlying soft tissue from pressure and/or shear.

Pressure Ulcer Prevention

Pressure ulcers cause long-term harm to the patient. These wounds place the patient at risk for not only local infection, but cellulitis, osteomyelitis, and sepsis. They increase length of stay, cause pain, and interfere with overall recovery. The IHI estimates that nearly 60,000 patients die each year from pressure ulcer complications.

Many pressure ulcers are preventable, but they remain common occurrences, affecting more than 2.5 million patients each year. Because of this, the IHI has developed guidelines in pressure ulcer prevention.

The work of pressure ulcer prevention has two major components:

- Identifying patients at risk
- Implementing preventive strategies for at-risk patients

═══════════════════════════*FAST FACTS in a NUTSHELL*

Please remember that you are the patient advocate. Through your experience and research you may discover an evidence-based practice not being used in your facility. Work to change that.

A. Conduct pressure ulcer (1) risk assessment and (2) skin assessment on all newly admitted patients and for those whose condition has changed. Document and report your findings as per facility guidelines. The Braden Scale (http://www.bradenscale.com/images/bradenscale.pdf) is the most common risk assessment tool used in the United States. It measures mobility, incontinence, sensory deficits, and nutrition/hydration status.

FAST FACTS in a NUTSHELL

> With any pressure ulcer risk assessment tool (or any risk-measurement device) you must also use your nursing judgment to determine skin alteration risk in patients whose risk is not reflected on the assessment.

B. Factors that place a patient at risk of developing pressure ulcers include:
  1. Advanced age
  2. Immobility
  3. Incontinence
  4. Insufficient protein and caloric intake
  5. Impaired cognition due to dementia, medication, or anesthesia
  6. Multiple comorbidities
  7. Circulatory abnormalities
  8. Dehydration
  9. Decreased blood supply to tissues caused by medical condition
  10. Use of medical devices that cause pressure to skin or bony prominences
C. Daily risk assessment for all patients should be employed to determine whether changes in mobility, incontinence, or nutrition/hydration have occurred.
  1. This allows for nurses to develop new interventions. Document and report findings as per facility guidelines
D. Complete daily head-to-toe skin inspection for at-risk patients.

FAST FACTS in a NUTSHELL

> Skin integrity can be altered within minutes.

  1. While performing a head-to-toe assessment, be sure to focus on areas of bony prominence, including the

sacrum, back, buttocks, heels, elbows, and those subject to device-related pressure or medical care, such as areas of oxygen tubing and masks, casts, splints.

2. Develop the habit of assessing the patient's skin at each interaction, such as when moving the patient from the bed to the chair or while turning and positioning, while toileting, or while assisting them with hygiene. Pay special attention to the sacrum, heels, back, buttocks, and elbows.

3. Ensure that all staff who care for the patient notify you of any skin alterations.

E. Keep the patient's skin dry and moisturized.

1. Clean incontinent patients immediately and at routine intervals.

2. Use only mild cleaning agents; soap dries the skin; avoid hot water.

3. Moisturize the skin with facility-approved emollients.

4. Perform or assist with daily hygiene.

5. Do not massage areas over bony prominences.

6. Do not allow perspiration, urine, stool, sputum, or wound drainage to remain on the skin for long periods.

7. If using diapers (although their use is discouraged) or absorbent pads, ensure that they keep the skin surface dry, are changed frequently, and that moisture barriers are applied to underlying skin.

FAST FACTS in a NUTSHELL

As with fall prevention, frequent rounds help to decrease pressure ulcers. During rounds you can do a skin check while repositioning the patient, apply a moisture barrier, toilet the patient, and offer food and fluids.

F. Ensure that the patient is receiving adequate nutrition and hydration.

1. Follow facility guidelines for requesting a dietician consult.

2. Encourage or provide adequate food and fluids, including prescribed snacks and supplements.
3. Monitor and report appropriate lab work, such as serum albumin, prealbumin, and transferrin.

G. Minimize pressure.
   1. Turn and position the patient frequently—a minimum of every 2 hours.
   2. Reposition patients in wheelchairs at least every hour. In alert patients, have them shift positions every 15 minutes.
   3. Use pressure-redistribution devices, such as pillows, cushions, or mattresses. Do not use doughnut-type devices in chairs or wheelchairs because they cause pressure areas on the skin.
   4. Raise the heels off of the bed.
   5. Keep the patient as active as possible to promote circulation. Consult physical therapy, occupational therapy, or, if in long-term care, the activity/recreation department.

FAST FACTS in a NUTSHELL

Protect the patient's skin when turning and positioning by using "draw sheets," "pull sheets," or other devices to prevent friction or skin tears.

Treatment of Pressure Ulcers

Nurses play an important role in the treatment of pressure ulcers, either as part of a wound-care team or in the direct care of the patient. The following is a general guideline for the care of pressure ulcers. As always, follow facility guidelines and policies regarding wound-care products and principles. The first step in treatment is to develop a comprehensive treatment plan and to ensure that all members of the health care team are following it. Then:

• Cleanse the wound as ordered.
• Assist with debridement and/or high-pressure irrigation.

- Use facility-approved dressings and supplies for each type of wound and treatment as ordered.

================= *FAST FACTS in a NUTSHELL*

Changing a dressing on any type of wound can be painful. Administer pain medication at least 30 minutes prior to changing the dressing. While providing care, determine whether the patient is experiencing pain. If so, discontinue wound care until the analgesic takes effect.

- Reassess the wound with each dressing change. Document and note progress of wound healing. Report to the MD if healing is not taking place or if the wound is worsening.
- Be alert for signs and symptoms of infection (drainage, foul odor, fever, high white blood cells, signs of sepsis, absence of healing) and report it.

================= *FAST FACTS in a NUTSHELL*

All pressure ulcers are colonized with bacteria. Routine cultures of the wound do not reveal the true contaminants of the wound bed. A wound biopsy may be necessary.

- Request a quantitative culture or tissue biopsy if the wound shows signs of infection or is not healing appropriately.
- Administer antibiotics as ordered.

Surgical Site Infection

The IHI estimates that 40% to 60% of surgical site infections (SSIs) are preventable. SSIs lead to increased length of stay, readmission, and increased morbidity and mortality. Many components are in place in health care facilities to prevent SSIs. If used consistently, they reduce or nearly eliminate preventable SSIs. These components include:

- Appropriate use of prophylactic antibiotics
- Appropriate preoperative hair removal
- Controlled postoperative serum glucose for cardiac surgery patients
- Immediate postoperative normothermia for colorectal surgery patients

Nursing interventions to prevent SSI include:

- Perform hand hygiene prior to assessing a dressing and/or removing old dressing material.
- Reduce airborne microorganisms by closing the patient room door and bedside curtains.
- Don clean gloves and remove the soiled dressing. Immediately dispose of old dressing material to avoid contaminating the clean dressing.
- Perform hand hygiene after removing old dressing material.
- Clean the surface where your new dressing material will be placed with facility-approved antimicrobial cleanser.
- Open and prepare sterile supplies.
- Cleanse the wound as ordered using ordered solutions. Be sure the solutions are not expired or have not been open for greater than 24 hours. "If in doubt, throw it out!"
- When cleaning a wound, clean from the area of least contaminated to most contaminated.
- Don sterile gloves when dressing a wound with sterile dressings.

10

Prevention and Treatment of Hip Fracture Along With Orthopedic Surgery Postoperative Care Tips

Patients with orthopedic conditions are cared for in a variety of health care settings and not just the hospital. Their immediate care could take place in a free-standing surgi-center, whereas their postoperative care could take place in the traditional hospital or at a subacute rehabilitation center. In any case, assessments and precautions are the same.

After reading this chapter, the reader will be able to:

1. List signs and symptoms of osteomyelitis
2. List signs and symptoms of hip fracture
3. List measures to prevent hip fracture
4. List nursing interventions in joint replacement surgery
5. List nursing interventions common in postoperative orthopedic cases

MUSCULOSKELETAL ASSESSMENT BACKGROUND

Your nursing assessment will not be as in-depth as that of a physician or orthopedic specialist. You will base much of your findings on observation of the patient while he or she attempts to ambulate or perform activities of daily living (ADL). You may also notice abnormalities during your care of the patient, such as while assisting with hygiene. You will also be guided by his or her chief complaint or immediate injury, should that unfortunate event occur while in your care.

A FOCUSED MUSCULOSKELETAL ASSESSMENT

Perform a focused musculoskeletal assessment when a patient complains of pain, tenderness, loss of function, or any abnormal sensation in muscles or bone.

Pain is the most common complaint in a patient with a musculoskeletal disorder. As with other conditions, the description of the pain will help to distinguish the source and type of disorder. Remember that pain is subjective and that individual and qualifying questions should be asked of the patient to ascertain the source of the pain. These include a description of the pain, its location, radiation, intensity, character, causative and relieving factors, action before onset of pain, body alignment of the patient, whether there is pressure on body surfaces (i.e., a cast on soft tissue). In general, pain described as:

- Dull ache may indicate bone pain
- Soreness or ache may indicate muscle pain
- Sharp and piercing can indicate fracture or an infection in the bone
- Being relieved by rest can indicate a musculoskeletal injury
- Increasing with activity and exercise can indicate joint or muscle damage

- Increasing over time can indicate an infection in the bone
- Radiating indicates that there is pressure on a nearby nerve
- Perform a skin assessment, noting any edema or color alteration such as cyanosis or mottling. Also note any signs of trauma such as bruises, lacerations, and cuts.
- Perform a neurovascular assessment of the affected extremity and compare to the unaffected side or to baseline. Alterations include pain, cyanotic skin, cool to touch, weakness, burning, numbness, and feeling of "pins and needles."
- Note any alterations in range of motion (ROM). ROM should be equal bilaterally. Can the patient move the affected part?
- Palpate pulse and compare to unaffected side. Also palpate the pulse distal to the injury. How does it compare to the unaffected side?
- Gently palpate the area of concern (bone, joint, or surrounding tissue/muscle). Note heat, warmth, cold, pain, edema, or tenderness.
- Ascertain whether the patient has any chronic health conditions, such as diabetes, pulmonary disease, cardiac disease, or previous musculoskeletal disorders.
- Note current medication use, including pain medication.
- Does changing position of the body or the affected limb cause pain or make the pain better?
- Ascertain when the complaint began and how long it has lasted. Is it getting worse?

COMMON MUSCULOSKELETAL CONDITIONS SEEN ON THE MEDICAL–SURGICAL UNIT

- Osteomyelitis
- Hip fracture
- Joint replacement
- Postoperative care of orthopedic patients

Osteomyelitis

Osteomyelitis is an infection of the bone and surrounding tissue. The infection can be caused by bacteria, virus, or fungus. It is difficult to diagnose, as the symptoms are variable and depend on the location of the injury and the overall health of the patient. Definitive diagnosis is achieved through x-ray, bone scans or magnetic resonance imaging, and blood cultures.

FAST FACTS in a NUTSHELL

Delayed recognition and treatment of osteomyelitis can lead to chronic infection, ongoing pain, loss of function, amputation of the affected limb, and death.

Osteomyelitis can occur from direct trauma to the bone, such as through surgery or fracture, from the blood spreading the infection from another site in the body, such as from a boil or upper respiratory infection or from contamination of open wounds, such as pressure ulcers or infected surgical wounds. Patients at risk of osteomyelitis include those with diabetes, the elderly, those with a history of blood-borne infections, obese patients, and those who abuse intravenous (IV) drugs. It is more difficult to heal in those patients who have a history of alcoholism, malnutrition, and liver disease.

Signs and symptoms of osteomyelitis include:

- A patient who has suffered a trauma to the femur or other long bone or who has had recent joint replacement; signs of infection include pain, redness, and drainage

FAST FACTS in a NUTSHELL

Osteomyelitis can occur from 30 days to a year or more after orthopedic surgery—be aware of the patient's surgical history.

- Pain is not a reliable symptom in patients with diabetes or pressure ulcers overlying the affected bone. These patients may not have pain. When there is pain it is described as constant throbbing that increases with movement.
- If the infection is blood borne, the onset is sudden and presents with septic signs and symptoms.
- If the infection has occurred due to a contaminated wound or a direct bone injury, there are no septic symptoms. The infected area is red, swollen, warm, and painful to the touch.
- The patient with chronic osteomyelitis has continuous drainage, pain, and swelling.
- Fever, generalized weakness, and malaise may or may not be present.
- Osteomyelitis of the vertebrae occurs in patients with a history of urinary tract infection or who abuse drugs.
- Note lab work, such as elevated erythrocyte sedimentation rate, leukocytes, and wound and blood culture results.

Nursing interventions include first the prevention of osteomyelitis:

- Preventing osteomyelitis involves communication between nursing and other health care professionals.
  - Elective orthopedic surgery should be postponed if the patient has an infection. If a current infection (i.e., urinary tract infection, cold, fever, etc.) is discovered during the admission process or preoperative check, or if the patient states history of recent infection, notify the surgeon and MD immediately.
  - Administer prophylactic antibiotics as ordered.
  - Obtain orders or follow facility guidelines to remove urinary catheters and surgical drains as soon as possible after surgery.
  - Follow aseptic technique when changing wound dressings and handling surgical drains.
  - Promptly report and treat wound infections.

Nursing interventions for those patients experiencing osteomyelitis include:

- Monitor the neurological status of the affected extremity. Report loss or change in sensation.
- Elevate the extremity if medically feasible.
- Assess for pain and administer pain medication as ordered and monitor for effectiveness. Report any increase in pain.
- Follow physician orders in restricting patient activity; however, attempt to promote independence and allow the patient to participate in ADL within the limits of his or her illness.
- Use gentle ROM for the affected extremity.
- Administer antibiotics and monitor for effectiveness.
- Monitor for signs of superinfection as an unexpected side effect of long-term antibiotic use (i.e., thrush, diarrhea).
- Prepare the patient for surgery, should it become warranted (to surgically debride the affected bone), if antibiotic therapy is ineffective.
- Use aseptic technique with all wound care.
- Promote a nutritious diet high in protein and vitamin C; encourage adequate hydration.

Hip Fracture

Hip fractures from falls are one of the leading causes of morbidity and death among the elderly. Unfortunately, falls occur within health care settings. The leading locations for falls are in the patient room and bathroom or while the patient is transferring from the bed to the chair. Several factors lead to patient falls in which the patient sustains a hip fracture. These include:

- Orthostatic hypotension caused by medication (antihypertensives, analgesics, sedatives)
- Impaired vision
- Lower limb dysfunction
- Neurological conditions
- Environmental hazards (poor lighting, slippery floor, unsafe footwear)

Types of hip fractures include:

- Femoral neck—the most common type in the elderly (most common in elderly women), most often associated with osteoporosis. Associated with mild trauma.
- Intertrochanteric—more often seen in male patients, associated with traumatic force.
- Subtrochanteric—more often seen in male patients, associated with traumatic force.

=== *FAST FACTS in a NUTSHELL*

If you find a patient on the floor after sustaining a fall, DO NOT move the patient. Complete your assessment where the patient lies. If you come upon the patient, do not leave the patient. Call for help.

Signs and symptoms of hip fracture include:

- One leg will be shorter than the other, adducted and externally rotated.
- If the fracture is displaced, there will be an obvious deformity.
- Bruising will be noted if the fracture is subtrochanteric.
- Unable to bear weight on the affected side
- Pain will be specific to the site of the fracture:
  - Femoral neck: groin and hip pain that increases with movement of the hip
  - Intertrochanteric: severe pain over the greater trochanter
  - Subtrochanteric: pain over the proximal thigh

Hip fractures may not be immediately evident, especially if the patient is unable to communicate or suffers from dementia. Be suspicious of a hip fracture if the patient has:

- Nonspecific leg, buttock, knee, thigh, groin, back, or hip pain/discomfort
- Difficulty bearing weight
- Bruising in the pelvic region

Nursing interventions for hip fractures include:

- As stated before, complete your assessment before moving the patient.
- Complete a set of vital signs, including head-to-toe assessment and neurological assessment.
- Assess for other injuries (cuts, scraps, or bruising).
- If there is a head injury or suspected head injury, notify the physician for follow-up evaluation (possibly head computed tomographic scan).
- Notify the physician and family of the fall.
- Prepare the patient for surgery.

Total Joint Replacement

Hip and knee replacements are the most common type of joint replacement.

The main nursing priority is to prevent complications, alleviate pain, and to promote mobility and return to an improved quality of life.

Nursing interventions for patients who have undergone joint replacement surgery include:

- Maintaining standard precautions, including hand hygiene
- Using strict aseptic technique when changing wound dressings or handling surgical drains
- Monitoring all drainage devices and ensure their functioning
- Documenting drainage characteristics, including amount and color; report signs of infection, including purulent, malodorous drainage
  - Infection in the operative site could be destructive, as the prosthesis may have to be removed and osteomyelitis may develop.
- Monitoring the surgical wound noting incision color, temperature of the skin surrounding the wound, swelling, redness, and loss of wound integrity
- Monitoring the patient for pain and administering analgesics; report a change in the character of the pain, especially

if the pain is deep, dull, or aching, which could indicate infection

- Monitoring vital signs and noting temperature increase or presence of chills
- Encouraging fluid intake and intake of a nutritious diet
- Maintaining the affected joint in proper alignment using an abductor pillow or as ordered
- Medicating the patient with prescribed analgesic prior to therapy or wound treatment in order to decrease pain and allow full participation in rehabilitation
- Turning and positioning the patient in bed using proper support to decrease pressure and prevent breakdown
- Monitoring the patient's skin and reporting areas of potential or actual skin breakdown
- Performing or assisting with ROM
- Encouraging participation in ADL

FAST FACTS in a NUTSHELL

Immediately report sudden increase in pain, change in skin color, change in temperature, loss of sensation, or shortening of the affected limb; all could indicate malfunction of the prostheses.

Postoperative Care of Orthopedic Patients

Patients who have undergone any type of orthopedic surgery and currently have a brace or cast are at risk for peripheral nerve dysfunction and vascular obstruction. Your interventions are aimed at maintaining function, sensation, and movement of the affected limb. Nursing interventions include:

- Palpate peripheral pulses, noting capillary refill, skin color, and temperature. Compare your findings with baseline and with the unaffected limb.
- Assess sensation in the affected extremity. Report increasing pain, numbness, or feelings of "pins and needles."

- Assess motion in the affected extremity. Report if the patient is unable to move the extremity on command, which may indicate nerve injury.
- Change in motion and sensation may also indicate altered circulation or dislocation of a prosthesis.
- Monitor vital signs reporting tachycardia or decreased blood pressure, both of which could indicate blood loss or decreased fluid volume.
- Monitor amount and characteristics of drainage on dressings and within drainage devices. Report abnormal increases and any other alterations.
- Note swelling of the operative area, which may indicate hematoma formation. Hematoma can place pressure on nerves and alter function and sensation of the extremity.
- Ensure that ordered stabilizing devices, such as abduction pillows, splints, and so on, are in place and in the correct position.
  - Ensure that devices are clean and dry and not stained with blood or drainage.
  - Perform frequent skin checks around and under the devices to ensure that there is no pressure causing altered skin integrity.
- Monitor patient for calf pain.

FAST FACTS in a NUTSHELL

Note that Homans' sign is not a diagnostic tool; an increase in unusual calf pain and inflammation should be reported.

- Check all dressings and casts frequently for drainage and bleeding. Be sure to check *under* the patient's affected extremity to ascertain whether drainage or blood has pooled.
- Observe for signs of bleeding and oozing from old puncture sites, or bruising following minor trauma. All could indicate altered clotting and should be reported.

- Administer intravenous (IV) fluids as ordered.
- Monitor lab work and report abnormalities in clotting studies and hematocrit.
- Administer anticoagulants as ordered. Monitor and report appropriate lab work.

Maintain intermittent compression stockings and devices. As with other patient equipment, ensure that they are in the correct place, functioning, and not placing undue pressure on the patient's skin.

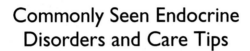

Commonly Seen Endocrine Disorders and Care Tips

Alterations in the endocrine system include investigating conditions of the thyroid, parathyroid, adrenal and pituitary glands, and pancreas; however, you will more commonly find alterations having to do with diabetes mellitus than any of the other conditions. This chapter focuses on two major alterations: hypoglycemia and ketoacidosis.

After reading this chapter, the reader will be able to:

1. List signs and symptoms of hypoglycemia
2. List nursing interventions of hypoglycemia
3. List signs and symptoms of diabetic ketoacidosis
4. List nursing interventions for patients with diabetic ketoacidosis
5. List nursing interventions for patients who have undergone thyroidectomy

ENDOCRINE SYSTEM ASSESSMENT BACKGROUND

The most common alterations you will see in the endocrine system have to do with diabetes. In the health care setting, you will usually know your patients who are diabetic, so you can develop your interventions and attempt to prevent hypo- and hyperglycemia. Hyperglycemia, or diabetic keto-acidosis (DKA), can occur as the *first* symptom of diabetes mellitus in those who are unaware that they have the disease. Known diabetics are at risk of hypoglycemia and hyperglycemia due to their concurrent illness. Part of your assessment is to ascertain the patient's knowledge base so that you can provide education for this patient in collaboration with the dietician and other staff.

A FOCUSED ENDOCRINE SYSTEM ASSESSMENT

A focused assessment will be based on the chief complaint of the patient or on the objective symptoms that you discover.

- Question the alert patient as to when abnormal signs and symptoms began.
- If the patient is complaining of pain, note onset, description, and location, and so forth.
- Note whether the patient has had or is experiencing an infection.
- Inquire about appetite changes, nausea, or vomiting.
- Obtain vital signs and note elevated temperature (hyperthyroidism); note respiratory rate and rhythm and blood pressure changes.
- Note and report abnormal lab results, including blood glucose levels and liver and thyroid function tests.
- Note complaints of weakness, fatigue, difficulty in ambulation, and muscle cramping.
- Note changes in voiding patterns, such as more frequent than usual.
- Note weight loss.

- Note excessive thirst.
- Note skin quality (turgor, dry, cracked, hot, or flushed).
- Note any complaints regarding sensory disturbances, such as numbness, tingling, weakness, or paresthesia.
- Note confusion, disorientation, or lethargy.
- Note signs of respiratory distress.

COMMON ENDOCRINE SYSTEM CONDITIONS SEEN ON THE MEDICAL–SURGICAL UNIT

- Postoperative care of a patient who has undergone thyroidectomy
- Hypoglycemia
- Diabetic ketoacidosis

Postoperative Care of a Patient Who Has Undergone Thyroidectomy

Partial or total removal of the thyroid is not a common surgery, so it bears mentioning so that you are aware of special postoperative precautions. Thyroidectomies are performed in order to remove cancer or to correct hyperthyroidism. If the removal is partial the patient may not have to take thyroid replacement medication. If the removal is total, the patient will be on replacement therapy for life.

Not only is the patient at risk for the "normal" complications of surgery, such as hemorrhage and infection, but he or she is also at risk for thyroid storm (severe hyperthyroidism, which can be fatal), tetany due to altered blood calcium levels, respiratory obstruction, laryngeal edema, and vocal cord injury.

When the patient is scheduled to arrive on your unit either postoperatively or after having been in the critical care unit, his or her room should be prepared:

- Include an emergency tracheostomy kit at the bedside
- Set up suction equipment
- Amps of calcium gluconate should be in the code/crash cart

Nursing interventions for those patients who have undergone thyroidectomy include:

- Monitor respiratory status—respiratory distress could indicate tracheal compression from edema.
- Auscultate breath sounds—accumulated secretions can cause rhonchi.
- Note dyspnea, cyanosis, and respiratory stridor; all of which could indicate laryngeal spasm, which is an emergency situation.
- The head of the bed should be elevated 30 to 45 degrees.
- The patient's head should remain in the "neutral position" in the immediate postoperative period. Encourage and assist the patient to not bend the head for several hours, or as ordered, after surgery. The head should be supported with pillows—this prevents tension on the surgical wound, which could produce edema.
- Assist the patient with turning/positioning and deep-breathing exercises.
- Suction oral secretions as needed, noting color and characteristics of the sputum.
- Check the neck dressing for blood and drainage frequently.

FAST FACTS in a NUTSHELL

Blood will pool posteriorly while the dressing will be dry anteriorly. While wearing gloves, feel behind the patient's neck on the pillow linen. Assist the patient in moving forward while checking the area behind or beneath the patient.

FAST FACTS in a NUTSHELL

The risk of bleeding is greatest up to 2 hours after surgery, but the risk continues for 24 hours postoperatively.

- Report patient complaints of being unable to swallow or unable to clear oral secretions. The patient may have edema.
- Provide humidified air in the patient's room to reduce discomfort and promote expectoration.
- If severe respiratory distress develops, prepare for emergency tracheostomy or a return to surgery.
- Keep communication with the patient simple, provide a pad/pencil as the patient should not speak in order to rest the vocal cords.
- Monitor vital signs and note elevated temperature, tachycardia, dysrhythmias, respiratory distress, and cyanosis.
- Report tetany, which is due to damage to the parathyroid and decreased calcium levels, which can occur 1 to 7 days after surgery—signs and symptoms are from neuromuscular irritability and include numbness, twitching, paresthesias, and seizure.
- Monitor calcium levels and report abnormalities.
- Monitor for pain and provide analgesics as ordered. Monitor their effectiveness.

Hypoglycemia

Hypoglycemia is one of the three major complications of diabetes. Hypoglycemia refers to a blood sugar level of less than 50 to 60 mg/dL. In a hospital setting, it can be caused by giving the patient too much insulin or oral hypoglycemic medication. Patients who have poor nutritional intake but are receiving their preadmission dose of insulin, and patients who are to receive "nothing by mouth" for a procedure or surgery are at risk for hypoglycemia.

Signs and symptoms of mild hypoglycemia (caused by surges in epinephrine and norepinephrine in response to the nervous system being stimulated) are:

- Sweating
- Tremors
- Increased heart rate; palpitations

- Nervousness
- Hunger
- Inability to concentrate
- Paresthesia
- Pallor
- Shakiness

Moderate hypoglycemia signs and symptoms include the prior-mentioned symptoms plus:

- Headache
- Irritability
- Lightheadedness
- Memory lapses
- Drowsiness
- Impaired judgment
- Slurred speech
- Numbness of the lips and tongue
- Double vision

Signs and symptoms of severe hypoglycemia (caused by severe central nervous system dysfunction) are:

- Severe disorientation
- Seizure
- Difficulty arousing from sleep
- Loss of consciousness

Nursing interventions include being aware of your facility's hypoglycemia protocols *prior* to an emergency. These are usually reviewed during orientation because they are a list of standing orders that nurses follow. You should be aware of the location of emergency equipment and drugs as well.

- Treatment ranges depend on the level of consciousness of your patient. For mild hypoglycemia, simply providing fruit juice or milk and retesting the blood sugar level in certain intervals will be all that is required. For moderate and severe levels, intramuscular and/or intravenous (IV) interventions are usually standing orders.

The most serious emergency for the diabetic patient is ketoacidosis. Although it accounts for a high rate of hospitalizations, it can occur in the already-hospitalized diabetic patient who is at risk. The three main causes of DKA include:

- Decreased or missed dose of insulin
- Illness/infection
- Undiagnosed or untreated diabetes (Many times this is the first symptom of DKA)

Because of an absence of insulin, there is an insufficient amount of glucose for the cells. To compensate, the liver increases its production of glucose. Both of these factors lead to hyperglycemia at levels greater than 250 mg/dL (can be as high as 300 to 800 mg/dL and greater depending on the degree of dehydration). The kidneys attempt to excrete the glucose and in doing so also excrete water and electrolytes. This polyuria (a patient can lose up to 6.5 liters of water in a 24-hour period) leads to dehydration. Fat breaks down into fatty acids and glycerol. The fatty acids are converted into ketones, which are acids now circulating uncontrolled in the bloodstream.

Those patients at risk for DKA are those diabetics who have or who are experiencing:

- Infection
- Myocardial infarction
- Pneumonia
- Stroke
- High physical or emotional stress
- Those receiving steroid therapy

Type 1 diabetics are at risk if insulin is missed and they have a concurrent medical issue. Type 2 diabetics are at risk if they are receiving medications such as corticosteroids and/ or have a concurrent medical issue.

> If your patient is diabetic and is to undergo surgery, has an infection, or whose oral intake is decreased, *notify the physician in order to obtain alternate insulin and blood glucose monitoring orders.* Do not alter or skip insulin administration.

Signs and symptoms of DKA include:

- Polyuria—excessive urination—one of the first signs of DKA
- Polydipsia—excessive thirst—one of the first signs of DKA
- "Fruity breath" due to excessive ketones—this is very characteristic of the condition
- Blurred vision
- Fatigue
- Flushed face
- Nausea/vomiting
- Abdominal pain—may be severe
- Muscle cramps
- Warm skin
- Tachycardia—due to dehydration
- Hypotension—due to dehydration
- Hyperventilation—deep, not labored breaths or Kussmaul respiration
- Shock—if dehydration is allowed to progress untreated
- Change in mental status—may range from alert, lethargic, to comatose
- Previously stated high blood glucose levels
- Arterial pH levels less than 7.30, serum bicarbonate less than 15 mEq/L and ketonemia
- Electrolytes are altered and may be high or low
- Blood urea nitrogen, creatinine, and hematocrit may also be elevated due to dehydration

Death can occur from cerebral edema and/or hypokalemia. Nursing interventions are aimed at correcting both dehydration and the hyperglycemia.

- Monitor and maintain the "ABCs": airway, breathing, and circulation.
- Frequently assess the patient's level of consciousness.
- Monitor fluid and electrolyte levels.

=== *FAST FACTS in a NUTSHELL*

Large volumes of IV fluid may be administered to correct the dehydration. Although correcting dehydration is a priority, be aware of fluid volume excess and overload.

- Monitor for signs of cerebral edema (headache, bradycardia, increased blood pressure, vomiting, and increased restlessness).
- Administer and monitor IV fluid—may initially include normal saline or ½ normal saline, then changed to 5% dextrose in water when blood glucose levels reach 300 mg/dL or less to prevent too much of a decrease in blood glucose.
- Monitor vital signs, noting changes in heart rate and blood pressure (tachycardia, hypotension).
- Monitor breath sounds, noting abnormal breath sounds indicating fluid volume overload.
- Monitor intake and output and kidney function tests.

=== *FAST FACTS in a NUTSHELL*

Ensure kidneys are functioning. Patients should have an output of at least 30 mL/hour. Ensure that the patient has adequate function prior to start of potassium infusions to prevent hyperkalemia.

- Monitor respiratory rate and pattern. If cyanosis or respiratory distress develops, the patient may develop respiratory arrest.
- Provide supplemental oxygen and monitor pulse oximetry.

- Obtain an order to insert and maintain a urinary catheter to accurately measure intake and output. Decreased or absent urine output can indicate altered kidney function. To decrease risk of infection, remove the catheter as soon as medically feasible.
- Monitor mental status frequently and report any abnormality.
- Monitor and report lab work that continues to be abnormal.
- Administer potassium as ordered.
- Administer insulin as ordered.
- Administer other medications as ordered.
- Ensure that there is a baseline electrocardiogram completed to compare to if the altered electrolytes cause cardiac dysrhythmias. If feasible on your unit, request that the patient receive cardiac monitoring, as he or she may have altered cardiac status due to hypokalemia/hyperkalemia.

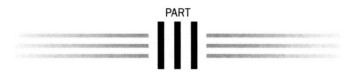

Must-Have Resources for the Medical–Surgical Nurse

12

Medical–Surgical Resources to Assist You in Your New Role

This chapter lists common resources needed by the medical–surgical nurse. Please refer to your facility's policy and procedures to supplement the information contained in this chapter. Included are helpful hints, a few "Oh, I remember that item," and snippets of hints from many different sources. This includes guides for proper syringe selection, pain scales and how to use them, intravenous (IV) solutions, common parameters for documentation purposes, fall prevention and restraint reduction, the "art" of intake and output, and weighing of patients and common calculations.

After reading this chapter, the reader will be able to:

1. Demonstrate use of enteral feeding calculation
2. List methods of fall prevention
3. Demonstrate measurement of edema
4. List measurement guidelines of syringes
5. Demonstrate Z-track method of intramuscular injection
6. List methods to reduce restraints

7. List correct use of pain scales
8. Demonstrate use of transmission-based precautions
9. Verbalize diagnosis of patient requiring intake and output measurement
10. List methods to prevent central line–associated bloodstream infections
11. Verbalize when and how patient should be weighed

ENTERAL FEEDING CALCULATION

For patients not on a fluid restriction and receiving less than a 100% solution (if not already premixed):

1. Change the percentage ordered to a decimal (i.e., 85% = 0.85).
2. Divide the total amount of formula by the decimal.
3. Subtract the original amount of formula from the total obtained.
4. Add water to the formula in the amount derived in Step 3.

Example: Calculate how much water to add to 240 mL of formula to make it a 25% solution.

Step 1. 25% = 0.25
Step 2. 240 mL / 0.25 = 960 mL
Step 3. 960 mL − 240mL = 720 mL

Answer: Add 720 mL of water to 240 mL of formula to make a 25% solution.

INTRAVENOUS CALCULATIONS

The use of electronic IV pumps is widespread in all institutions. Their use is to ensure that IV fluid infuses within the ordered time frame, to prevent fluid overload, and correct administration of medications. Many IV pumps calculate the drip rate and pharmacies premix ordered solutions. In order to maintain patient safety, however, IV drip rates should be rechecked by the nurse prior to starting the IV fluid.

$$\text{Hourly rate: mL/hr} = \frac{\text{total infusion (mL)}}{\text{hours of infusion}}$$

Minute flow rate (drops per minute mL/hr $\times$ drop factor / 60 minutes = drops/min)

FALL PREVENTION

Injuries from falls are "never events" because they are associated with high rates of morbidity and death. The Institute for Healthcare Improvement (IHI) has included injuries from falls among its Partnership for Patients topics. Falls can be prevented by:

- Completing the facility fall screening on admission and following facility guidelines for reporting the results and need for consultations
- Being aware that, in addition to the fall-risk assessment, you must use your nursing judgment to determine whether a patient is at risk of falling. The patient may score a "not at risk" on the form, but in actuality, fall precautions should be put in place.
- Ensuring patient rooms are free of clutter and walkways are clear
- Ensuring the patient is wearing his or her eyeglasses and hearing aids
- Ensuring the patient wears nonslip footwear at all times
- Ensuring that lighting is adequate in patient rooms and halls; use nightlights
- Ensuring the call bell is in the patient's reach at all times
- Ensuring personal care items are within reach of the patient at the end of each patient encounter
- Keeping the bed in the lowest position with brakes locked; include this action in your documentation
- Locking wheelchair wheels; include this action in your documentation
- Ensuring that personal alarms, such as those in the chair and bed, are turned "on"; include this alarm check in nurses' notes

- Promptly investigating any alarms (call bells, personal, and so on)
- Ensuring all ambulatory and other assistive devices are in working order
- Never leaving a patient alone in the bathroom
- Instructing all patients to call for assistance prior to ambulation or transfer
- Performing patient rounds at least every 1 to 2 hours or as facility guidelines dictate; inquire whether the patient needs to use the bathroom; place personal items, call light, and phone within reach; turn and position the patient if necessary; and last, inquire whether the patient needs any other assistance
- Personalizing fall-prevention strategies for each of your patients
- Placing patients at greatest risk for fall nearer to the nurses' station or provide one-on-one observation
- Using protective equipment, such as hip protectors, as per facility guidelines
- Being aware of patients' medications that may increase their fall risk, including sedatives, antihypertensives, hypnotics, and pain medication

MEASUREMENT OF EDEMA

Measure pitting edema by pressing a finger firmly for several seconds (and releasing) over the shin. 1+ pitting = 2 mm, 2+ pitting = 4 mm, 3+ pitting = 6 mm, and 4+ pitting = 8 mm.

VITAL SIGNS

- **Pulse Strength**—When documenting the strength of a pulse measurement, the following scale is used:
  - 0 = absent or not palpable
  - 1+ = the pulse is diminished or barely palpable
  - 2+ = a normal pulse strength

- 3+ = full pulse or increased
- 4+ = a bounding pulse
- **Blood Pressure Hints**—Normal adult blood pressure < 120/80.
  - Normal systolic < 120; normal diastolic < 80
  - Prehypertension: systolic = 120 to 139 or diastolic = 80 to 89
  - Stage 1 hypertension: systolic = 140 to 159 or diastolic = 90 to 99
  - Stage 2 hypertension: systolic ≥ 160 or diastolic ≥ 100
  - Blood pressure readings should not be based on a single reading completed in one arm. If an abnormal reading is found using an electric or automatic cuff, retake it with a correctly fitting manual cuff.
  - Obtain a manual blood pressure reading *only* in the following disease conditions: irregular heart rate, peripheral vascular obstruction (i.e., blood clot), shivering, seizure, excessive tremors, inability to cooperate, and a previous blood pressure less than 90 mmHg systolic.

===*FAST FACTS in a NUTSHELL*

Speaking to the patient immediately prior to or having the patient speak while you are taking his or her blood pressure can increase the reading.

- **Measuring Temperature**—Normal adult temperature range is 96.8° to 100.4° F. Core temperature is the most reliable indicator of body temperature.
  - Average oral/tympanic: 98.6° F (tympanic is one site of core body temperature)
  - Average rectal: 99.5° F (another site of core body temperature)
  - Average axillary: 97.7° F (usually 1 degree lower than core)
  - Hypothermia below 96.8° F
  - Pyrexia (fever) 100.4° to 104° F
  - Hyperthermia is temperatures greater than 104° F

FAST FACTS in a NUTSHELL

The patient may demonstrate a temperature less than 98.6° F hours before a patient "spikes" a temperature or feels ill. Recheck all low-temperature readings with another thermometer at a core site (rectal or tympanic).

SYRINGE SIZE SELECTION

Choosing the correct syringe and needle size is imperative in order to prevent nerve or bone damage, pain, and inadvertent medication injection into a vein or artery.

- Subcutaneous injection (sub-q)–for administration of 0.5 to 1 mL of medication.
  - Needle size: 27 to 25 gauge, 3/8" to 5/8"
  - In an average-size adult, a 25-gauge 5/8" needle can be inserted at a 45° angle
  - A 25-gauge ½" needle can be inserted at a 90° angle
  - In a thin patient, a sub-q injection can be inserted into the upper abdomen

FAST FACTS in a NUTSHELL

For a sub-q injection, if you can grasp 2" of tissue, insert the needle at a 90° angle; if you can grasp 1" of tissue, insert the needle at a 45° angle.

Subcutaneous insulin: Use an insulin syringe only.

- Intradermal—Used for skin testing, such as tuberculosis and allergy tests.
  - All injections are inserted at a 5° to 15° angle with the bevel of the needle up.
  - Use the inner forearm or upper back (allergy testing) for easy visualization.

- Intramuscular—Use for administration of 2 to 3 mL of medication.
  - The size of the needle, the body profile (thin, normal, or obese), and the amount of medication to be injected should correspond to the site of the injection in the adult.
  - Needle size: 2- to 22-gauge 1"–1 ½"
  - All injections are inserted at a 90° angle.

Sites for IM injection include:
- Vastus lateralis: Allows for rapid drug absorption.
  - In very thin patients, the muscle should be grasped during the injection to lift the muscle away from the bone.
  - This site is more often used in children.
- Deltoid: Easily accessible. Used for small amounts of medications or when other sites are inaccessible.
  - Most often used for immunizations in adults; however, the danger to radial, axillary, brachial, and ulnar nerves as well as the brachial artery is present.
- Ventrogluteal: The *preferred, safer site* in adults as it is away from major nerves and blood vessels and is usually a large muscle (Figure 12.1).
  - Can be used for large-volume, irritating medications. Easily identified by using bony landmarks.

THE Z-TRACK METHOD OF INTRAMUSCULAR INJECTIONS

The Z-track method is used in IM injections in order to minimize skin irritation, decrease the occurrence of lesions, decrease pain at the site, and to prevent the injected medication from leaking from the injection site.

- After drawing up the medication to be administered, change the needle to remove irritating medication from the needle shaft.
- Select the injection site and cleanse the skin using the facility-approved method.
- Pull the skin overlying the injection site 1" to 1 ½" laterally to the side.

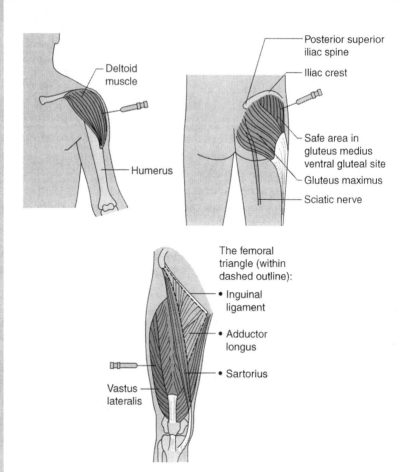

FIGURE 12.1 Sites for intramuscular injection.

- While holding the skin taut with your nondominant hand, inject the needle.
- Aspirate for blood return. If there is no blood, inject the medication slowly.
- Leave the needle in place for 10 seconds (allows medication to dispense).
- Withdraw the needle and release the skin.

REDUCING USE OF RESTRAINTS

It has been found that the use of restraints in fall prevention can actually *cause* serious life-threating injuries and even death. Follow facility guidelines for obtaining a restraint order. Know the policies and procedures on your units for restraint use. Nurses can reduce the use of restraints by:

- Using facility-approved methods to reduce fall risk (i.e., personal alarms, or monitored bathroom visits)
- Managing confusion and delirium (activities, maintain current level of orientation with visible cues, verbal explanations, and reminders)
- Promoting sleep (quiet environment)
- Improving nutritional status
- Optimizing medication use
- Managing pain
- Promoting functional status
- Modifying physical environment and equipment (use of low beds, better lighting, skid-proof slippers, transfer assistive devices, "crash pads"/mats around the bed)
- Promoting mobility and exercise (refer to physical therapy/occupational therapy for gait and balance consultation, and strength building), provide own wheelchair for unit mobility
- Providing regular toileting
- Providing a comfortable bed and promoting optimal positioning

INTRAVENOUS SOLUTIONS

Isotonic Solutions

- Dextrose 5% in water (D5W)—to supply water for the body, to correct increased serum osmolality

- 9% sodium chloride or normal saline (NS, 0.9% NS, 0.9% NaCl)–to replace large sodium losses
- Lactated Ringer's—used to correct dehydration, sodium depletion, and replacement of GI fluid losses

Hypertonic Solutions—Dextrose-containing solutions are used to correct dehydration, hyponatremia, to administer medications, for short-term nutrition, and to correct hyperkalemia

- Dextrose 10% in water (D10W)
- 3% to 5% sodium chloride (3% to 5% NS, 3% to 5% NaCl)
- Dextrose 5% in 0.9% sodium chloride (D50.9% NaCl, D50.9% NS, D5NS)
- Dextrose 5% in 0.45% NaCl sodium chloride (D50.45% NaCl, D50.45% NS, D5 ½ NS)
- Dextrose 5% in lactated Ringer's (D5LR)

Hypotonic Solutions—Used to hydrate stable patients receiving total parenteral nutrition or tube feedings

- 0.45% sodium chloride (half normal saline, z NS, 0.45% NS)
- 0.33% sodium chloride (⅓ NS)

PAIN SCALES

No pain assessment scale is definitive, as they are based on the subjective experiences of the patient. As the nurse, use measurement tools, but also value the input of family members and caregivers in order to give you insight into the patient's usual responses.

Both the patient *and* the nurse must understand how pain scales are administered for accurate, reliable results. The patient must be taught the pain scale to be used and this must be documented. The correct pain scale based on the patient's cognitive level must be used for accurate assessment.

- **Numeric Rating Scale**—A 0 to 10 scale with "0" as no pain and "10" as the worst pain ever experienced. Each number must be explained so that the patient can give an accurate response.
  - 0 = no pain
  - 1 = mild pain that does not interfere with activities of daily living (ADL)
  - 2 = minor annoying pain
  - 3 = pain is noticeable and occasionally distracting; ADL possible
  - 4 = moderate pain that may distract from an activity
  - 5 = moderately strong pain that can't be ignored; ADL still possible with effort
  - 6 = moderately strong pain that interferes with ADL
  - 7 = severe pain that interferes with ADL and sleep
  - 8 = intense pain, ADL severely limited, patient able to speak with great effort
  - 9 = excruciating pain; patient unable to perform ADL or speak; moaning/crying
  - 10 = unspeakable pain; bedridden and possibly delirious
- **Verbal or Descriptive Scale**—The patient describes his pain as "no pain" to "mild," "moderate," "severe," or "pain as bad as it could be."
- **FACES Pain Scale–Revised**—The Wong–Baker pediatric scale as revised for adult use. Please note that the *patient* is taught to point to the face that best describes how he feels. The nurse is not to assume the patient's pain level based on what he "looks like."
- **Pain Assessment in Advanced Dementia**—The PAINAD Scale (http://www.geriatricpain.org/Content/Assessment/Impaired/Documents/PAINAD_Tool.pdf). The PAINAD scale (Pain Assessment in Advanced Dementia) is used in patients who are cognitively impaired and are unable to communicate their pain. Items measured are breathing, negative vocalization (moaning, groan, calling out, crying), facial expression, body language, and consolability.

TRANSMISSION-BASED PRECAUTIONS

Transmission-based precautions are the second tier in infection control. The first tier is Standard Precautions used for all patients. It is based on the assumption that all patients have the potential to pass on a blood-borne illness or infectious disease. Follow Centers for Disease Control and Prevention and facility guidelines for specific guidelines.

- **Airborne Precautions**
  - Patient should be placed in a private room with negative airflow.
  - All who enter the room should wear a respirator or facility-approved mask.
  - This type of precaution is appropriate for patients with measles, chickenpox, disseminated varicella zoster, and pulmonary or laryngeal tuberculosis.
- **Droplet Precautions**
  - Patient should be placed in a private room or cohorted with a patient with the same illness.
  - All who enter the room should wear a mask when closer than 3 feet from the patient.
  - This type of precaution is appropriate for patients with influenza, mumps, and parovirus B19.
- **Contact Precautions**
  - Patient should be placed in a private room or cohorted with a patient with the same illness.
  - All who enter the room should wear gloves and gowns.
  - This type of precaution is appropriate for patients with wounds colonized with multiple-drug resistant organisms; herpes simplex; *Clostridium difficile;* and incontinent patients with hepatitis A and Shigella. Those patients with impetigo, scabies, and pediculosis should also be placed in contact isolation.

Visitors and family members of the patient in isolation should be taught about hand hygiene as well as donning, removing, and disposing of personal protective equipment. This teaching should be documented in the nurses' notes as well as whether they follow precautions as taught.

INTAKE AND OUTPUT—A LOST "ART"

Unfortunately, measuring intake and output (I&O) has somehow fallen by the wayside, with nurses thinking it only needs to be completed when ordered. Nurses need to understand that I&O is one of the main tools we have to ascertain kidney function and hydration status in the patient. A nurse can initiate I&O on any patient for whom he or she feels it to be necessary, and an MD may place an order for *strict* I&O. Any hospitalized patients experiencing the following medical conditions are at increased risk for fluid-volume deficit and should have an I&O measured.

- Chronic renal disorder
- Chronic cardiac disorder (i.e., heart failure)
- Receiving IV therapy
- On a fluid restriction
- Dependency on others for nutrition and hydration
- Fever
- Vomiting, diarrhea, or both
- Receiving diuretics
- Immediate preoperative patient
- 24 hours postoperative or postprocedure (follow facility guidelines)
- An unstable medical condition
- Receiving enteral nutrition
- Receiving "nothing by mouth" for any reason
- Nasogastric tube for suction
- Indwelling urinary catheter

- Drains or suction
- Colostomy
- Severe trauma/burns

If it seems like every patient on a medical–surgical unit should have I&O completed...you're right.

FAST FACTS in a NUTSHELL

Ice chips are measured as ½ the original amount; for example, 100 mL of ice is equal to 50 mL of fluid. All foods that are liquid at room temperature should be included in an I&O record (i.e., ice cream, gelatin).

Other I&O Hints

- If a patient is receiving enteral feedings, the water used to flush the tube should be counted as intake.
- All parenteral fluids, such as piggybacks and blood, should be counted as intake.
- Know your facility policy on "zeroing out" an IV or feeding pump at the start/end of your shift for total volume measurement.
- When emptying a Foley at the end of your shift, remove the urine from the tubing well (allowing it to drain into the collection bag) to obtain the total amount.
- Use a urimeter for accurate I&O for those patients on strict I&O.
- Incontinence of stool and urine must be measured by estimation and number of times a diaper or pad had to be changed.
- Colostomy drainage is counted as output as is vomit.
- Wound drainage is counted as output.
- Always follow standard precautions when obtaining output and draining collection devices.

- Explain the importance of obtaining accurate I&O measurements to the patient and his or her significant others.
- Communicate to other staff (especially those reporting to you) the importance of accurate I&O. Ensure that they are educated in how to obtain I&O measurements prior to delegating the task.

HOW TO CALCULATE TRUE URINE

Patients receiving genitourinary irrigation (continuous bladder irrigation [CBI]) must have "true urine" obtained when measuring their I&O. This is the amount of irrigant minus the urine amount and is calculated as total amount of irrigant infused–the total amount of output. The difference in amount is the true urine (1,000 cc of CBI − 1,200 cc output of urine = 200 cc of true urine).

PREVENTING CENTRAL LINE–ASSOCIATED BLOODSTREAM INFECTIONS

Central line use is becoming more prominent on the medical surgical unit, in both subacute and outpatient settings. Although central line use allows for long-term venous access, it is also a portal for bacteria and fungi to enter directly into the bloodstream. This can lead to severe sepsis and death. According to the IHI 90% of central–line associated bloodstream infections (CLABSIs) occur with central lines. They also estimate that there are 82,000 central line-associated bloodstream infections and up to 28,000 central line infection-associated deaths every year.

The IHI in partnership with such organizations as the Association for Professionals in Infection Control and Epidemiology and The Joint Commission, have developed strategies to reduce these deadly infections. They created a group or "bundle" of evidence-based interventions that, when implemented, together prove to have a better patient outcome. See the complete "how-to guide" at www .ihi.org. Components of the bundle include:

- Hand hygiene
- Barrier precautions
- Chlorhexidine skin antisepsis
- Optimal catheter site selection and avoiding the femoral vein
- Daily review of line necessity and prompt removal when no longer necessary

Follow your facility guidelines for the insertion precautions and use and monitoring of central lines.

WEIGHING PATIENTS

The patient's weight is a key indicator as to his or her fluid status. It must be completed correctly, however, in order to be a useful assessment tool. Remember that for every 2.2 pounds of weight gained or lost, one liter of fluid is retained or lost.

- The patient should be weighed at the same time each day, preferably in the morning prior to eating and drinking and after using the restroom.
- The same equipment should be used to weigh the patient each time.
- Daily weigh-ins can help to indicate whether fluid is being gained due to heart failure.
- Baseline weight should be obtained on admission and maintained throughout the admission.

Bibliography

Arora, V., & Johnson, J. (2006). National patient safety goals: A model for building a standardized hand-off protocol. *Joint Commission Journal on Quality and Patient Safety, 32*(11), 646–655.

Black, J. M., & Hawks, J. H. (2009). *Medical–surgical nursing clinical management for positive outcomes* (8th ed.). St. Louis, MO: Saunders Elsevier.

Boushon, B., Nielson, G., Quigley, P., Rutherford, P., Taylor, J. Shannon, D., & Rita, S. (2012). *How-to guide: Reducing patient injuries from falls.* Cambridge, MA: Institute for Healthcare Improvement. Retrieved from http://www.ihi.org

Clark, C. (2013). Civility can be learned! *Reflections on Nursing Leadership, 39*(3).

Department of Health and Human Services, Office of Inspector General. (2010). *Adverse events in hospitals: National incidence among medical beneficiaries* (OEI-06-09-00090). Washington, DC: Author.

Doenges, M. E., Moorhouse, M. F., & Murr, A. C. (2006). *Nursing care plans guidelines for individualizing client care across the life span* (7th ed.). Philadelphia, PA: F. A. Davis.

Hammerschmidt, R., & Meador, C. (1993). *A little book of nurses' rules.* Philadelphia, PA: Hanley & Belfus.

Hartford Institute for Geriatric Nursing. Geriatric Resource Nurse. (2012). *Age-related changes in health.* Retrieved from http://www.nicheprogram.org

Hartford Institute for Geriatric Nursing. Geriatric Resource Nurse. (2012). *Falls.* Retrieved from http://www.nicheprogram.org

Hartford Institute for Geriatric Nursing. Geriatric Resource Nurse. (2012). *Pain*. Retrieved from http://www.nicheprogram.org

Hartford Institute for Geriatric Nursing. Geriatric Resource Nurse. (2012). *Pressure ulcers and skin tears*. Retrieved from http://www.nicheprogram.org

Hartford Institute for Geriatric Nursing. Geriatric Resource Nurse. (2012). *Restraints*. Retrieved from http://www.nicheprogram.org

Hartford Institute for Geriatric Nursing. Geriatric Resource Nurse. (2012). *Urinary incontinence*. Retrieved from http://www.nicheprogram.org

Health-care Associated Infections (HAIs). (n.d.). Retrieved from http://www.health.gov/hai/prevent_hai.asap

Horgas, A. L. (2012). Assessing pain in older adults with dementia. *Try this: Best practices in nursing care to older adults* (D2). Retrieved from http://www.consultgerirn.org/uploads/File/trythis/try_this_d2.pdf

Institute for Healthcare Improvement. (2011). *How to guide: Prevent adverse drug events by implementing medication reconciliation*. Cambridge, MA: Author. Retrieved from http://www.ihi.org

Institute for Healthcare Improvement. (2011). *How to guide: Prevent catheter-associated urinary tract infections (CAUTI)*. Cambridge, MA: Author. Retrieved from http://www.ihi.org

Institute for Healthcare Improvement. (2011). *How to guide: Prevent pressure ulcers*. Cambridge, MA: Author. Retrieved from http://www.ihi.org

Institute for Healthcare Improvement. (2012). *How to guide: Prevent central line-associated bloodstream infections (CLABSI)*. Cambridge, MA: Author. Retrieved from http://www.ihi.org

Institute for Healthcare Improvement. (2012). *How to guide: Prevent harm from high-alert medications*. Cambridge, MA: Author. Retrieved from http://www.ihi.org

Institute for Healthcare Improvement. (2012). *How to guide: Prevent harm from venous thromboembolism (VTE)*. Cambridge, MA: Author. Retrieved from http://www.ihi.org

Institute for Healthcare Improvement. (2012). *How to guide: Prevent injuries from falls and immobility*. Cambridge, MA: Author. Retrieved from http://www.ihi.org

Institute for Healthcare Improvement. (2012). *How to guide: Prevent surgical site infections*. Cambridge, MA: Author. Retrieved from http://www.ihi.org

Institute for Healthcare Improvement. (2012). *How to guide: Prevent ventilator-associated pneumonia*. Cambridge, MA: Author. Retrieved from http://www.ihi.org

MacReady, N. (2013). Student nurses report shoddy infection control practices. *American Journal of Infection Control, 2013*(41), 760–763.

Mandal, A. (2014). *Oxygen theraphy administration.* Retrieved from http://www.news-medical.net/health/Oxygen-Therapy-Administration.aspx

Noah, P. (2004). *Neurological assessment: A refresher.* Retrieved from http://www.modernmedicine.com/modern-medicine/news/neurological-assessment-refresher

Potter, P. A., & Perry, A. G. (2006). *Clinical nursing skills and techniques* (6th ed.). St. Louis, MO: Mosby Elsevier.

Potter, P. A., & Perry, A. G. (2009). *Fundamentals of nursing* (7th ed.). St. Louis, MO: Mosby Elsevier.

Reilly, R. (2008, August 11). Are you a good mentor? *Nursing Times .net.* Retrieved from http://www.nursingtimes.net/are-you-a-good-mentor/1795628.article

Salmon, N., & Constantine, L. (2004). *Focused cardiovascular assessment.* Retrieved from http://w3.rn.com

Shuttleworth, A. (2004). Teaching nurses the importance of microbiology for infection control. *Nursing Times.net, 100*(36), 56.

Smeltzer, S. C., Bare, B. G., Hinkle, J. L., & Cheever, K. H. (2008). *Brunner & Suddarth's textbook of medical–surgical nursing* (11th ed.). Philadelphia, PA: Lippincott Williams & Wilkins.

The Studer Group. (2007). *Hourly rounding supplement.* Pensacola, FL: Sacred Heart Hospital.

Walsh, D. (2010). *The nurse mentor's handbook: Supporting students in clinical practice.* Berkshire, England: McGraw-Hill, Open University Press.

Index